Books by Danice Sweet

Floating Zoo and the Whale Motel

Consider It Joy

I Will Speak Your Name

He Makes Me Laugh

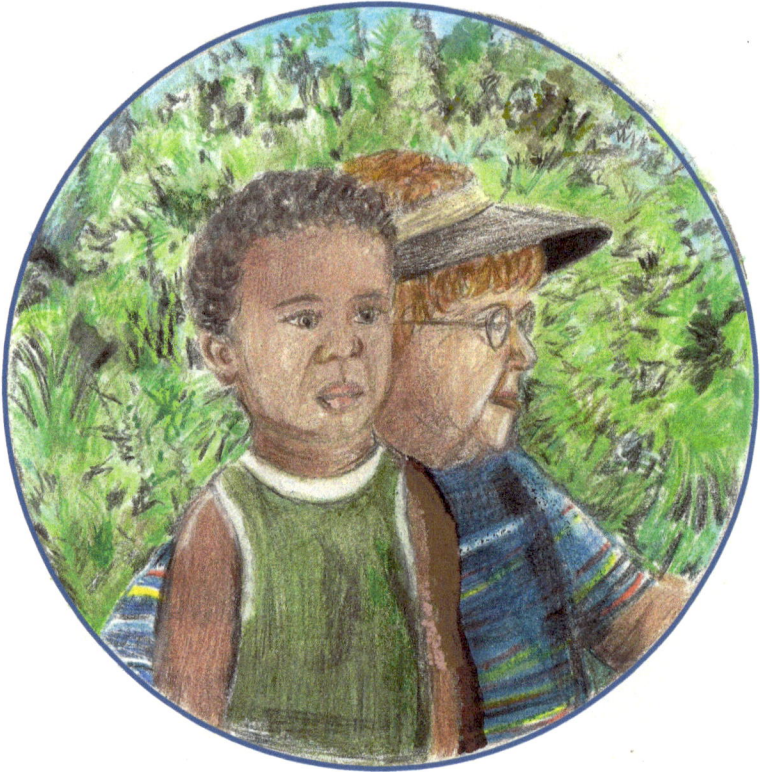

Music CD included with book purchase.

To receive your recording of author Danice Sweet and her group, Revival, singing her songs which she discusses in this book, fill out this coupon and mail it to the address below.

PLEASE PRINT

Name: _____

Street Address: _____

City, State, Zip Code: _____

MAIL TO:

Pearson Publishing Company
555 N. Shoreline Blvd., Suite 104
Corpus Christi, Texas 78401

Gloria Won!

A Journey of Faith through A.L.S.

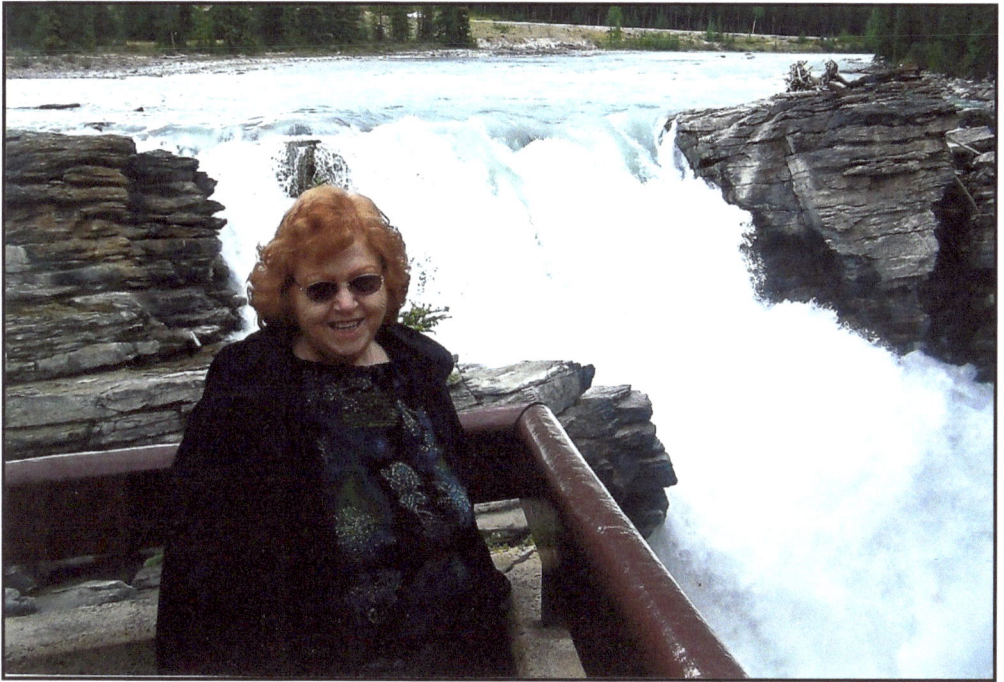

By Danice Sweet & Dr. Gloria Clover

Pearson Publishing Company
Corpus Christi
2011

Library of Congress Control Number: 2011922290

ISBN-13: 978-0-9843326 -8-7   perfect bind

ISBN-13: 978-0-9843326-9-4   e-book

Cover photo: Chet Sweet
Cover design: Katherine Pearson Jagoe Massey
Book design: Katherine Pearson Jagoe Massey and Danice Sweet
Cover production: IDS Consulting
Photo on title page: Danice Sweet

Published by
Pearson Publishing Company
Corpus Christi, Texas
www.PearsonPub.US

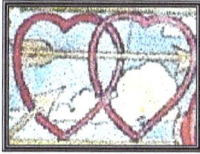

Contents

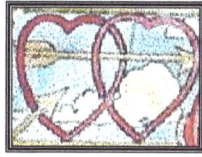

Foreword

This book reveals the journey of one woman and her experience with ALS or Amyotrophic Lateral Sclerosis, also known as Lou Gehrig's Disease. It is not meant to be anything other than that. Everyone's situation is different. Each person is affected by ALS in different ways. The treatment discussed in this book is not endorsed by anyone or validated by any medical organization.

Our prayer is that this helps you on whatever journey you or a loved one are on. This road is not an easy one. Nothing rewarding ever is easy. My momma taught me that.

The words in italics are Mom's. The others are mine.

Danice Sweet
December 2010

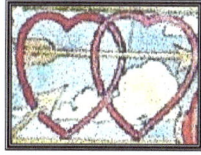

Special Thanks

I'd like to thank all the family, friends, students and parents of students who shared their memories of Gloria Clover. I'm also so grateful to my lifelong friend and sister in Christ, Donja Hayes Cary, for proofreading and editing and inspiring me to keep on keeping on.

Danice

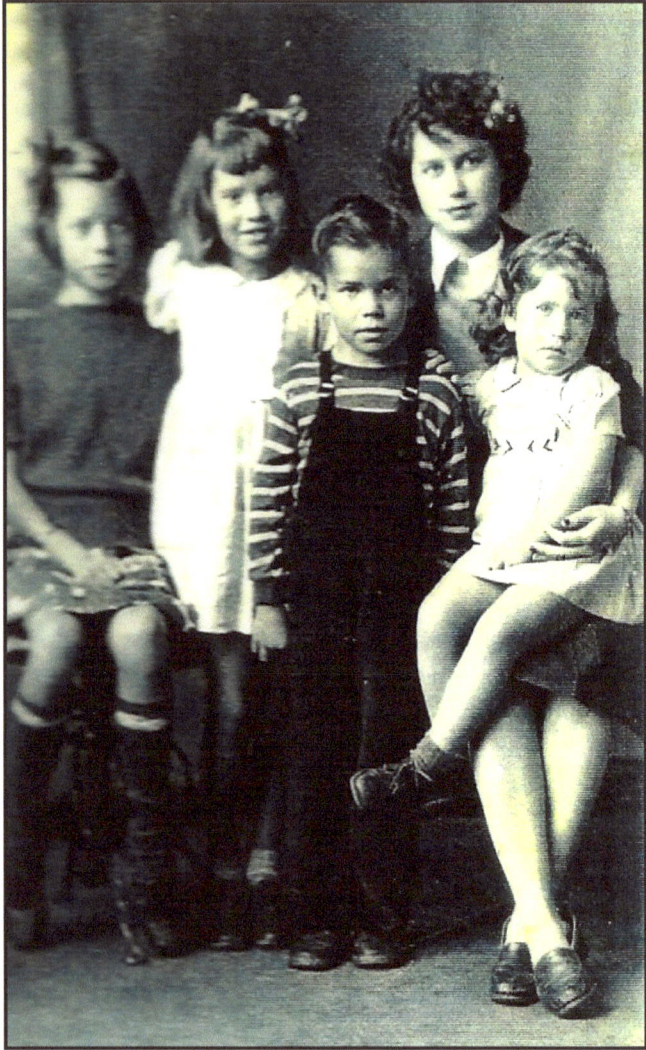

From left to right: The youngest five siblings are Aunt Gerry, Aunt Evelyn, Uncle Tom, Aunt Jeannie and Mom on her lap.

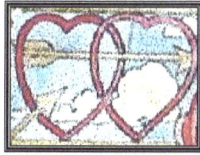

Chapter One: The Youngest

My mother was the youngest of ten children. She grew up in Wagoner, Oklahoma, not far from Tulsa but even closer to Muskogee. She was a red-headed, freckle-faced, bright young woman who loved her family, loved the Lord, and enjoyed competition. She kept a journal for a good part of her life and edited her own writings into notebooks. She used these for resources to help her remember everything from someone's birthday to what Christmas gifts she had given, or what vitamins she took. These journal articles are included with her permission in this book.

I remember my grandfather, George Washington Hardy, as a man who was soft-spoken, liked strong coffee, thick like syrup, and played the harmonica while wearing a poncho like a Mexican blanket. His skin was the color of butterscotch from working outside all his life. When we arrived from Kansas to visit, he would reach into his pocket and pull out two quarters, so we could walk through the backyard to the Safeway and buy M&M's. We thought we were big stuff walking through the grass to the alley, past the laundry drying on the line, on to the neighborhood grocery store with money our grandpa had given us.

Mom's mother, Elizabeth Hardy, didn't smile often, but when she did you remembered it. She liked to fish and play dominoes more than anything. We came to visit one weekend, and she wasn't at home. She was down at the Fish Dock. I had never seen anything like it. All these older folks were sitting in lawn chairs inside a metal building that floated on top of a lake. In the metal building was a huge square hole. All these old folks had buckets, and their fishing poles were stuck in the huge square hole in the water. It smelled awful like dead fish and dirty worms. I remember when walking in, Grandma seeing Mama, and all of us doing our best not to fall in while trying to keep the floating dock level. She just smiled. She didn't set her pole down or stop fishing, but she smiled.

Mom loved retelling the story of when her parents were fishing on a little boat. Her mother lost her balance and fell on the minnow bucket and crushed it. Her father could not contain himself and laughed until he hurt. I have such a clear picture of that in my mind and love the thought of them both having a laugh. I didn't see that too often, perhaps because mostly the only times time the whole family got together was at funerals.

Grandma Hardy kept butter rum flavored Lifesavers in the door of the refrigerator, where butter should be, in case her "Sugar Diabetes" went low. If I'd only known then, what those Lifesavers would mean to me now. Being diabetic and taking three shots a day, I understand just a glimmer of what she went through. Now we're so blessed to have disposable syringes, and insulin pens, and sugar free everything.

I reckon by the time your tenth and last child has her last child nothing is really that impressive. That last child of the tenth was me. Being a redheaded, freckled-faced kid, everyone always rubbed my head, but I especially recall my grandpa loving my hair. While sitting on the floor, I remember looking up at my grandparents sitting side by side on the couch. Sometimes Grandpa would be singing songs about sinking ships while Grandma was busy in the kitchen washing dishes and preparing the next meal. I guess that's why I always felt the need to try harder, to sing louder, to write more. I wanted my folks to be proud. I wanted my grandparents to look down from Heaven and smile.

I wrote a song several years ago called *I've Got A Father*, inspired by my mother's love for her dad.

I've got a Father
We've got a Father
Always tried to be home early not late
Didn't want to see the look on Daddy's face
When I walked through the door
And he'd been waiting on me
You see I wasn't afraid of any punishment
Just couldn't stand the thought I'd disappointed Daddy
One more time
And put a tear in his eye
You see he's the kind of father always hoped for the best
He was there for me when everyone left

Chorus:
And I've got a Father
Don't want to let him down
He's got a faith in me
Farther than I can see
His love for me abounds
He's got plans and dreams
Of what he wants me to be

And I don't want to disappoint Daddy
'Cause I know he loves me

One day I'm going to make it to that heavenly gate
Can't wait to see the look on God's face
When I kneel down before
My one and only Lord
He'll wrap His arms around me, I'll climb on His knee
Put my hand on His shoulder, breathe a sigh of relief
At home I'll be
Eternally
You see He's the kind of Father never let me down
He's prepared for me a home and a crown

Repeat Chorus

Bridge:
A long time ago a boy left home
Spent all the money he would ever own
Came to himself ready to give up
Then he pictured home and his father's love
Repeat Chorus
I've got a Father
We've got a Father
You've got a Father
Don't want to let Him down

Mom loved her niece, Dee. In fact, since they were close in age, they were more like sisters. The last ten years or so, Mom would occasionally call me Dee and even call my husband Chet by Dee's first husband's name, Tony. She would stop herself and apologize, but I realized it was truly a compliment because she and Dee were that close.

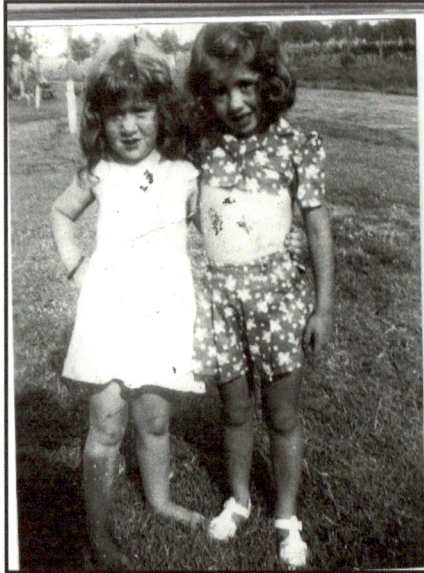

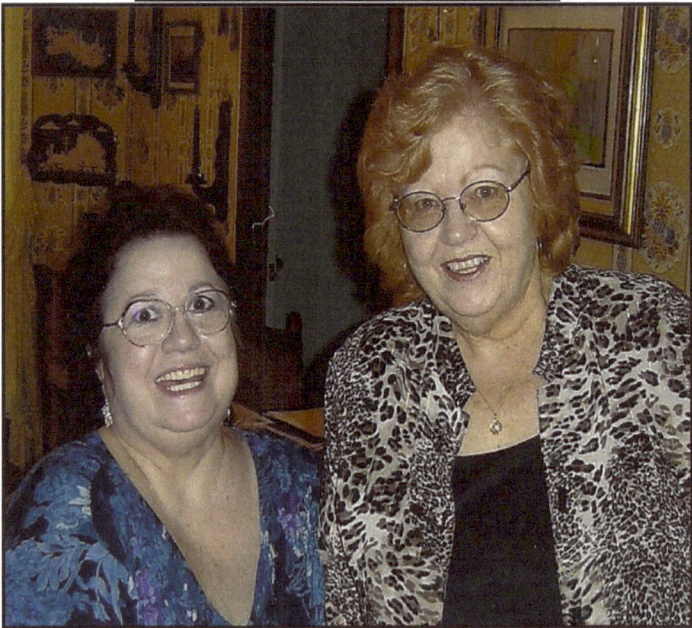

Gloria and Dee   Dee & Gloria

I love both of these pictures. Dee just called yesterday to check on me to see how I was holding up. She was such a dear friend to Mom that it brings me comfort to hear her voice.

One of my favorite stories Dee told in front of Mom last summer was that when they were teenagers, Dee had received a love letter from her boyfriend, who ended up being her first husband, Tony. Mom was driving and wanted to read what the letter said so badly she couldn't stand it. She ended up driving off the road and into someone's white picket fence trying to read over Dee's shoulder in the car. Mom turned red and grinned when she heard Dee tell the story, so I presume it to be true.

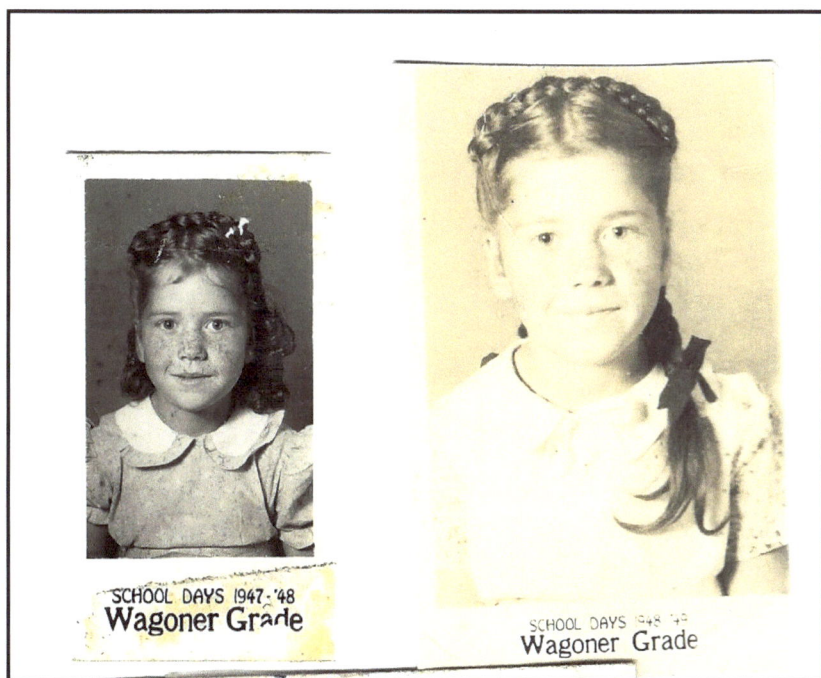

Gloria at ages 7 and 8, in her school pictures from Wagoner, Oklahoma.

Being the last of the Hardy family, I'm sure there were comparisons made between Mom and her brothers and sisters especially when it came to their education. It was always stated that you did the very best you could in school. Anything less than an "A" was not acceptable. I think I may have heard that a time or two as well. Mom would work on papers before they were due, and when the teacher or professor decided the class didn't have to do the paper, Mom would be disappointed. I believe I received some of that trait.

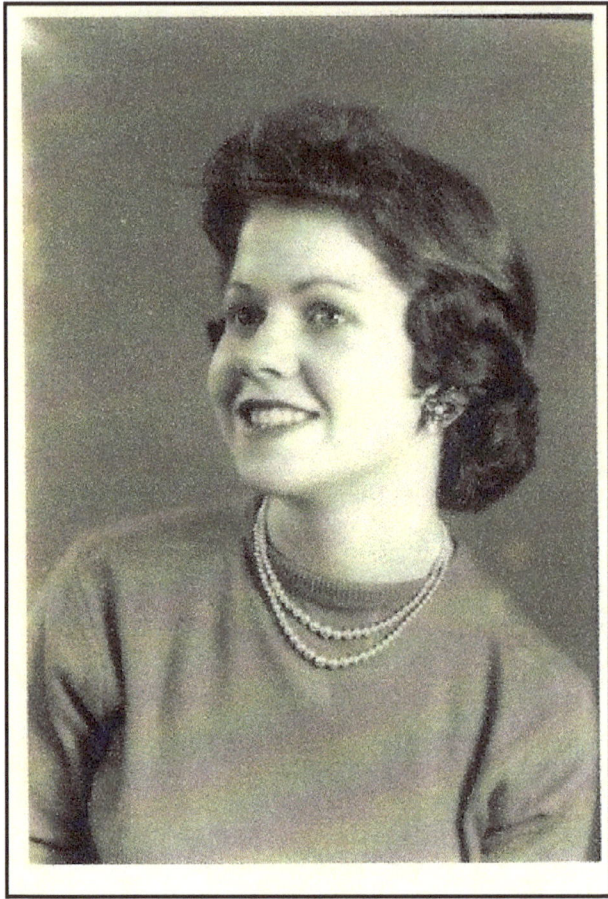

Mom's Senior Picture from High School

In school Gloria excelled. She was heart-broken when her parents moved three times during her senior year. She said she would cry herself to sleep crying loudly enough so she knew they could hear her. She never felt at home at school after her family moved from Okay, Oklahoma. There she had played on the girls basketball team, played steel guitar, and was to be the valedictorian. What a sad thing it was for her to have to move to Newkirk, Oklahoma. Working at Albright's was what she did to keep her mind off the loss of the friends and activities she so desperately missed.

at Albright's--Newkirk, Ok.
dating Jacob (Jake) Paul Clover.

In high school she was a member of the basketball and softball teams, Oklahoma Honor Society, Band "Okettes", cast of Junior Play. She was also secretary of her 4-H club and Junior Class. In college, Gloria was a member of the German Club, Annual Staff, Drama Club, Pep Club and school newspaper staff.

Mrs. Clover is a member of the Newkirk Church of Christ and was married to Jacob Paul Clover on January 1, 1962. Clover is employed at Mauer-Neuer at Arkansas City. She is the daughter of Mr. and Mrs. George Hardy of 517 West 7th, Newkirk. She has 7 sisters and 2 brothers. Her hobbies include bowling, swimming, skiing, horseback riding, badminton, writing and poetry.

Employed as secretary to Mrs. Irene Foxworthy, Mrs. Clover's duties include maintenance of various records and other secretarial tasks.

Whether you desire to open a savings account with Albright's, or have need for any of the other services offered by the company, each of Albright's 46 employees are well qualified to assist you and welcome the opportunity to be of service.
—pd. adv.

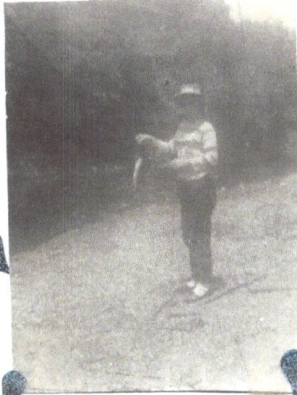

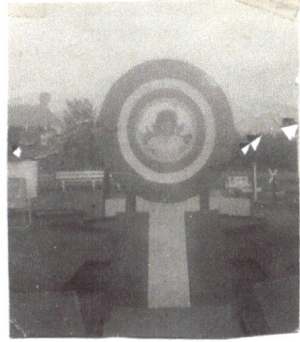

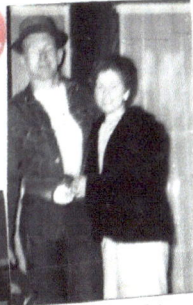

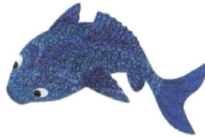

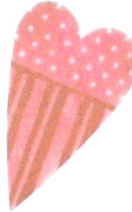

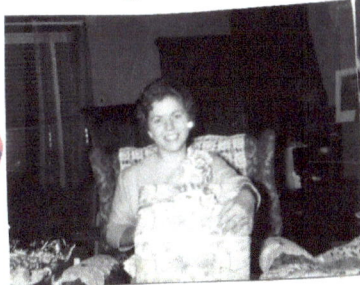

1-21-1962

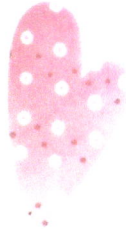

Wedding Shower

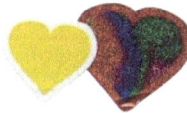

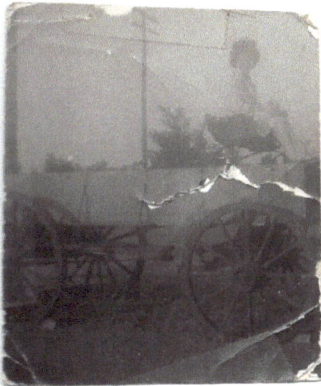

This is one of the scrapbook pages Mom put together. I love that the article on the top left corner says that her hobbies, "include bowling, swimming, skiing, horseback riding, badminton, writing and poetry."

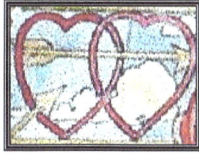

Chapter Two: A Wife

We decided to get married on January 1st, 1962. I was 21, he was 23. I told him I wouldn't marry someone that wasn't a Christian even though I wasn't a baptized believer myself. He agreed to this and we were baptized very early in the morning at Newkirk, Oklahoma by the Church of Christ preacher.

Later that day we drove to Sedan, Kansas and we were married by the Church of Christ preacher at Sedan, Kansas with his wife present. The preacher read the wedding ceremony from a book and called us Shirley and Bill which must have been the last two names he had penciled in his wedding ceremony book. We were too nervous to correct him.

We never did receive our marriage certificate and wondered if he'd sent in the wrong names. About 40 years later, Jake gave me a framed copy of our certificate that he had managed to get. We had been legally and officially married after all.

I know what I know about being a wife from my mother. Her priorities were always her God, her husband, her children, and family and friends, pretty much in that order. We were always fed, clothed, encouraged, and loved.

I'm sure it was a challenge to be a Christian wife in the 1960's. I know it was tough to make ends meet, and that Mom and Dad lived in an upstairs apartment on North A Street in Arkansas City, Kansas. I pass that apartment every week on my way to Roosevelt School. I don't know what hopes and dreams they had as a young married couple. I hope most of their dreams came true.

Our house was never fancy, but it was neat and clean. The first week of every month the first drawer of every shelf or drawer was organized. The second week of every month the second drawer of every shelf or drawer was organized and so on.

The Message Bible states in Proverbs 31 that "a good wife is hard to find, and worth far more than diamonds, she has these characteristics,... First thing in the morning, she dresses for work, rolls up her sleeves, eager to get started. She senses the worth of her work, is in no hurry to call it quits for the day....she's quick to assist anyone in need, reaches out to help the poor....when she speaks she always has something worthwhile to say, and she always says it kindly...."

I'm not surprised that this description sounds like Gloria Clover.

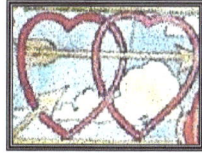

Chapter Three: A Mother

Our first home was an apartment in Ark. City. We have lived there off and on ever since. Our two daughters, Dayna and Danice, were both born there.

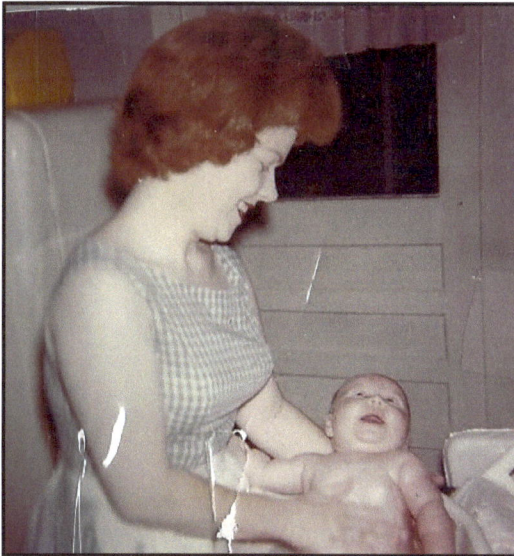

Things were tough in rural Kansas, but they were about to get tougher. When my sister was two months old, my parents and my sister were involved in a horrible car accident. A man fell asleep and crossed the yellow line hitting them head on, on a two lane highway in Oklahoma. All three Clovers were in the hospital. My sister was not expected to survive because her head ended up under the gas pedal. Not only did she survive, but she thrived! I was born eighteen months later and have heard the stories told of that accident my whole life. The retelling varies with each person, but the worn and faded newspaper clipping tells quite a story.

I don't know if Mom underlined parts of it or was marking out what wasn't true.

Dayna wasn't expected to make it through the night. My grandmother was determined to get the blood out of the little newborn outfit Dayna had been wearing. She prided herself on being able to get a stain out of anything. Mom said that she scrubbed that little dress until her hands were raw. Perhaps that was her way of coping with the situation and the heartache.

Four Are Injured In 3-Car Crash

A three-car collision at the intersection of U. S. 77 and S. H. 51 three miles south of Orlando injured four persons Sunday night.

Jake P. Clover, 24, Kansas City, Mo., his wife and a week-old daughter were injured. None was believed to be serious.

The accident occurred when Fay Howe, 50, Buffalo, attempted to turn into U. S. 51 striking the Clover's vehicle and forcing it into another car, Trooper Lee Elyson said.

... was only slightly injured.

Clover Family Is Improving

A recent report on Mr. and Mrs. Jacob Clover and their two month old daughter, Dayna Elizabeth, who were injured in an accident south of Orlando, Okla., March 31, indicates all are improving.

The baby was discovered to have a broken leg and possibly a broken arm, Clover has no broken bones, but the doctor says he may need a long time to recuperate from the force of impact of being thrown out of the car. Mrs. Clover is no longer a patient but is helping care for her husband and daughter.

Their address is Baptist Memorial Hospital, Oklahoma City, for those wishing to send cards.

3-31-63

3 Residents Are Injured

Jacob Clover Family In Oklahoma City Hospital

Mr. and Mrs. Jacob Clover and their two-month-old daughter, Dayna Elizabeth, 1225 N. Eighth St., are receiving treatment in an Oklahoma City hospital for injuries received in a two-car accident Sunday three miles south of Orlando, Okla., at the intersection of U. S. 77 and S. H. 51.

First treated at Perry Memorial Hospital, the baby later was rushed to Oklahoma City, with a highway patrol escort, where a brain specialist was waiting to treat her. She had received possible head injuries and bone fractures and was in a semi-conscious condition.

Clover, 24, received undetermined neck, back and arm injuries, underwent extensive X-rays, and was later transferred to Oklahoma City. Mrs. Clover, 22, is reported much improved from a head laceration.

The Clover family was traveling north in a pickup truck with the baby in a seat between them, when a car driven by Fay Howe, 50, an oil field worker moving from Buffalo to Bristow, made a left hand turn in front of them, according to the patrol. Howe sustained rib injuries and was not listed as in serious condition.

The Clovers moved from Newkirk to Arkansas City about a year ago and the baby was born here. Clover works for Maurer-Neuer. While living at Newkirk several years, he worked for Albright's.

Mrs. Tony Roberts, 204 North C St., a niece of Mrs. Clover, and Mr. Roberts, drove to Perry to see the injured family Tuesday night. The baby and her father were later moved to Oklahoma City. Mrs. Roberts says she has received no further word from the Clovers.

Baby, 3 Others I... Collision

Three members of an Ark... City, Kan., family, including infant girl, and a man m... from Buffalo to Bristow we... tients Monday in Perry Mem... hospital with injuries re... shortly before 7 p.m. Sunday... miles south of Orlando at th... tersection of U.S. highway... state highway 51.

Still undergoing X-ray... other examination was Da... Elizabeth Clover, two m... old. She was in a semi-c... scious condition with head... juries and possible bone fractures.

Improving and receiving... ment for head injuries be... not serious was her father, ... Clover, 24, Arkansas City... wife and the child's mother... la Ann Clover, 22, was muc... proved with a laceration ... forehead.

Fay Howe, 50, an oil field... er moving from Buffalo to B... tow, sustained rib injuries ... was improving and not list... serious condition.

The Clover family had ... traveling north in their au... bile on U.S. 77. Howe ... going south on 77 in a p... truck and was preparing to ... a left turn onto SH 51 whe... vehicles collided.

Bill Edwards, Orlando ... chief, made a run to the a... dent scene with the Orla... resuscitator to aid Da... Elizabeth, who developed t... ble breathing after the ac... dent. However, it wa... necessary to use the ox...

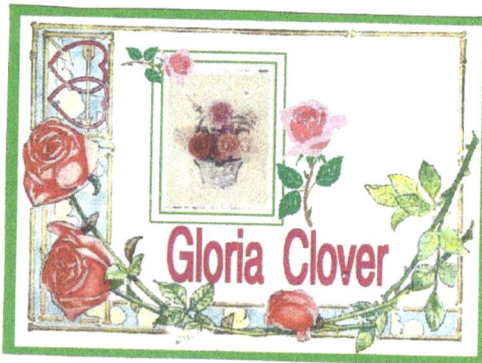

Gloria Clover

THE SICK: The Clovers are still in the hospital at Okla. City. Word was received from them today (Tuesday), they are better. They are thankful for the car's and letters, and for the gift from several of the congregation.

12

My sister surprised everyone. Dad had received neck, back, and arm injuries, and Mom had a sprained wrist and head lacerations. Dayna was diagnosed with "Accident-Induced Cerebral Palsy." Her little leg was put in a cast at two months old. The doctor set the cast wrong causing her right foot to land wrong when she started walking. Her right arm and right leg did not function as well as the left side. She had another surgery when she was twelve years old to try to fix the first surgery. They waited until they thought she had achieved most of her height.

She told me that she had planned to go shopping at a mall in Wichita, Kansas after the cast from the repairs was removed, but she was in far too much pain to do so. Last week, after going through the antique trunk my mother once hid in as a child, I found my sister's cast.

Dad had worked at Maurer -Neuer Packing plant and since Mom was the least injured from the accident, she asked the supervisor at the plant if she could go to work instead, and she did. She still says it was the worst job she had ever had or seen in her life. She never would eat hot dogs after that. Ever.

They had dear friends at the time, Fred and Nancy Woods. Mom wrote in a journal that,

"They would cheer Dayna on as she tried to stand and then learned to walk. Their encouragement was amazing."

I'm not certain when the fire occurred. Mom was pregnant with me, and Dayna was one year old, consequently that would be around 1963-1964. A vaporizer caught fire, and I know Mom and Dad lost almost everything.

A couple, Don & Norma Cole, came by from the church and asked them what they needed. What do you say when you need everything? Don and Norma brought a freezer full of beef. They became wonderful, life-long friends, always there for my folks in good times and bad.

I guess I was a bit of a surprise when eighteen months later I came along. Dad finally went to work back at the meat packing plant. He eventually became a government meat inspector and began working in Emporia, Kansas.

I have fond memories of Emporia, such as good friends, great church family, and swinging on our swing set with my sister. We would look up at the clouds and find shapes in them like dragons and puppy dogs.

My Mom and Dad always raised us both to try our best and never give up. I learned to ride my bike on Eighth Street, and my sister was riding behind me not long after.

In the early 1970's, we lived in the college town of Emporia, Kansas. A few days before one Halloween, Mom got into an accident while driving. She was dressed as Colonel Sanders from the Kentucky Fried Chicken franchise or KFC as they are known today. Three long-haired hippies got out of their car, probably high on more than just "life," and they apologized for not signaling at the intersection. However, when the police arrived, their story changed. They asked why some crazy redhead dressed as Colonel Sanders would be trusted, and why they weren't taken at their word. I remember Mom coming home very frazzled.

We had a list of chores on the refrigerator door with a list of different chores for each day of the week. I don't remember what the consequence was for not doing the chores. I didn't know there was an option.

I do remember getting my mouth washed out with soap for being disrespectful. The reason I remember it so well, was the only soap left in the house was Lava soap. If you are not familiar with Lava soap, it was a hand cleaner primarily for men who worked in grease. It was gritty and did not have a good flavor. One mouth washing was enough for me.

We learned to skate in Emporia, Kansas when I was in second grade. My sister was determined she would skate too, and she did. We started bowling, and yes, again, with her left arm swinging, my sister and I became state doubles champions. Mom and Dad bowled on leagues regularly.

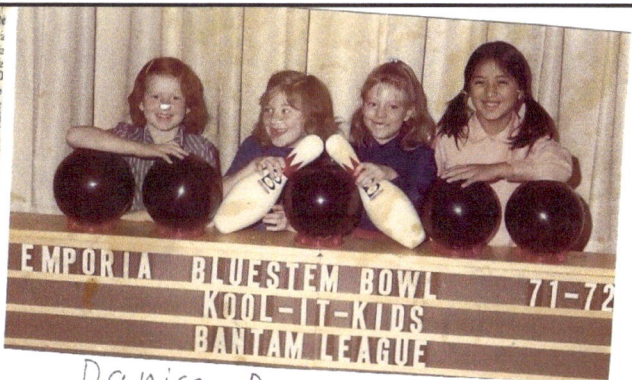

EMPORIA BLUESTEM BOWL   71-72
KOOL-IT-KIDS
BANTAM LEAGUE

Danice   Dayna

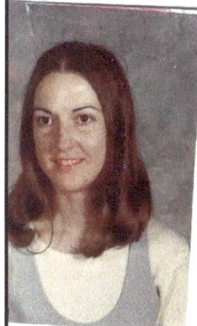

s. Erickson
nice's Teacher

... nours
re spent i
... owling a
Emporia and

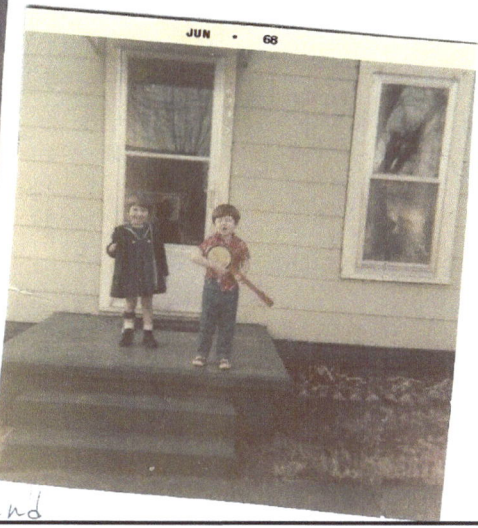

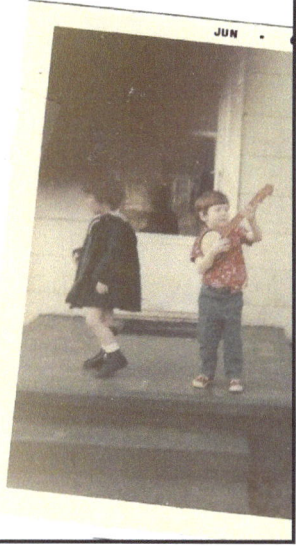

JUN · 68

JUN ·

This is another one of the scrapbook pages Mom put together. Dayna and me on the front porch of our house on Eighth Street in 1968; Dayna and me in our Bowling Years 1971-72 in Emporia, Kansas; and Ms. Erickson my favorite teacher from second grade.

We eventually moved back to Arkansas City, but Mom traveled back and forth to Emporia to complete her teaching degree. I remember being shocked to hear she had received a speeding ticket while driving her little red Volkswagon.

We said the word "bored," one summer. What a mistake! My sister and I said, "We're bored, Mom." Mom's frustration was completely evident as she replied, "Bored? There's a list of chores for each of you on the fridge; you are in art camp, swimming lessons, and have the time to do anything your hearts' desire; and you are bored? I'd like for you to wipe down all of the baseboards in this two story house. If you are still bored after that, I will find something else."

We cleaned baseboards for two days, on our knees, and never said we were bored again. In fact, a few summers ago, Mom called and said, *"I'm getting close to the B word."*

I replied, "Which B-word?"

She said, *"You know the one.....Bored!"*

So we got together and went shopping.

She was a coupon clipper. Even the grandkids recall Mom giving them a stack of coupons, sorted by which aisle they were in, and sent down the row of the grocery store. Always looking for a bargain.

I never heard the word handicapped when it came to my sister. It was always assumed she could do anything she set out to do, and she did. She is an incredible person and a loving mother to three amazing children and a precious grandmother to her two grandsons. They call her Grandma Dayna, and they call Mom, Grammy. I am called Ne-Ne, which has slid into Nini.

My life would be incomplete without the joy her children have brought to all of us, especially Mom. When my sister found out she was expecting her first child, my mother started shopping. I recall a knitted Santa Claus bib mom found at a craft fair, that her first grandchild, Chrissy, had to have. It was not really practical, but cute none the less.

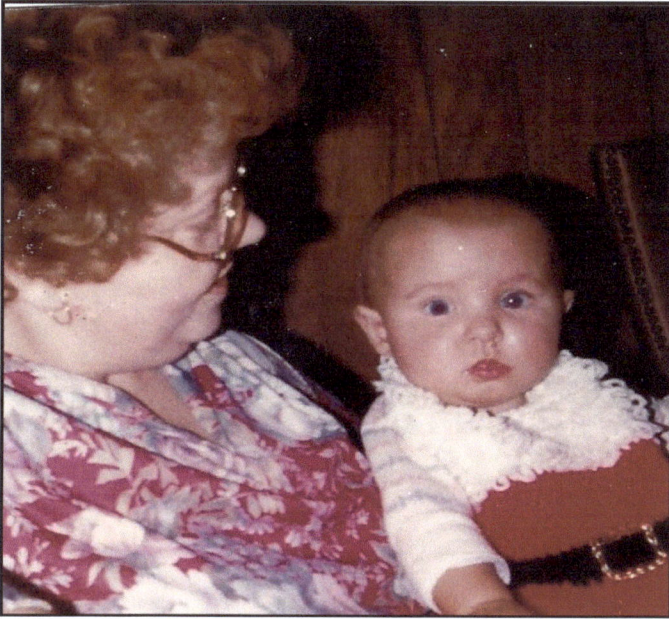
Mom and Chrissy at Christmas

Christmas at our house was amazing! Being the youngest of ten children, Mom believed that everyone should have ten presents each to open on Christmas Eve. That was our tradition.

"Loved the holidays, particularly Christmas. Hope my children and grandchildren always value family and get together regularly. Make Christmas, 4th *of July, Easter, Thanksgiving, and Memorial Day special by getting together and observing traditional celebrations/remembrances. Remember each others' birthday and realize and appreciate how special each one is." (Checklist, 2008)*

She started working on buying Christmas presents for the next year the day after Christmas was over. She beamed as we went around the room, someone always wearing the elf hat and handing out one gift at a time, in an organized fashion so that you could see everyone's face when each gift was opened.

The pile of presents under the tree was like a small forest of other trees around it. The gifts would flow over into other rooms and tables. There was no way you could compete with her giving. It was impossible.

There were always special friends with us at each holiday. Mom wanted to be certain every friend, widow, or neighbor had a place to go.

Aunts, cousins, family friends, ladies from church, and young people were always welcome in the Clover home.

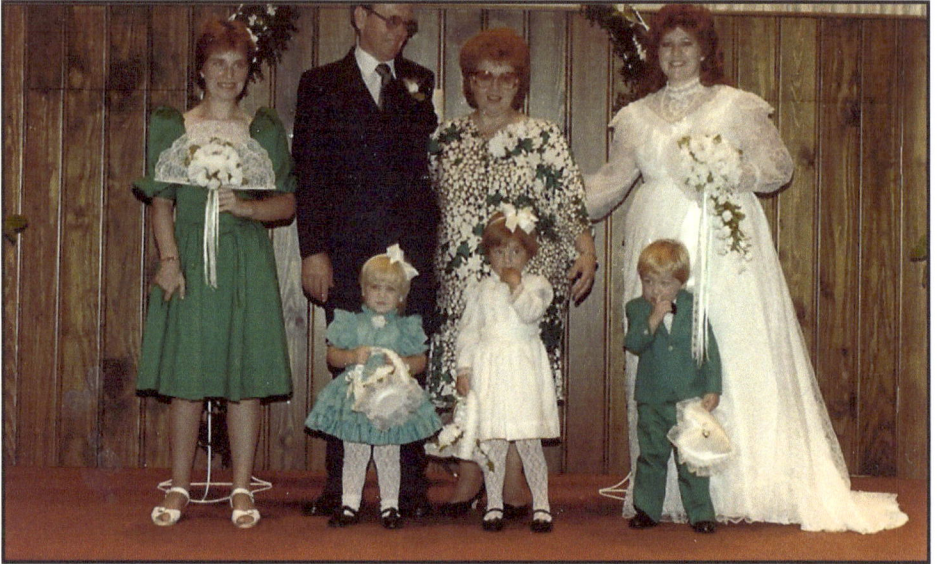

Mom loved her children, grandchildren and especially her great-grandchildren. She helped to raise Dayna's kids, as they moved back into our family home when all three were in diapers.

Christine Elizabeth-She loved animals from an early age. When she was little she had a twinkle in her eye. She still loves animals.
Lucas Dale- He helped his Grandpa Jake work on cars, trucks, etc. from an early age. He's always been fascinated with vehicles and driving.
Holly Elayne- She was the most outgoing of the three and loved to go on trips with her Aunt Danice and her group Revival. She was always a good student and took making good grades seriously. (Checklist, 2007)

When her great-grandsons came along, it was love at first sight. She doted on them. Their yard looked like a park with toys, slides, wagons, a horse-shaped tire swing and lastly a helicopter-shaped jungle gym. At Christmas time you could not compete with her gift giving. You just tried to keep up. She always had a gift drawer. She would gather presents, perfume, crafts and special things she knew people collected so she would always have a gift on hand for any special occasion. We all became accustomed to bringing a few extra gifts without names on them.

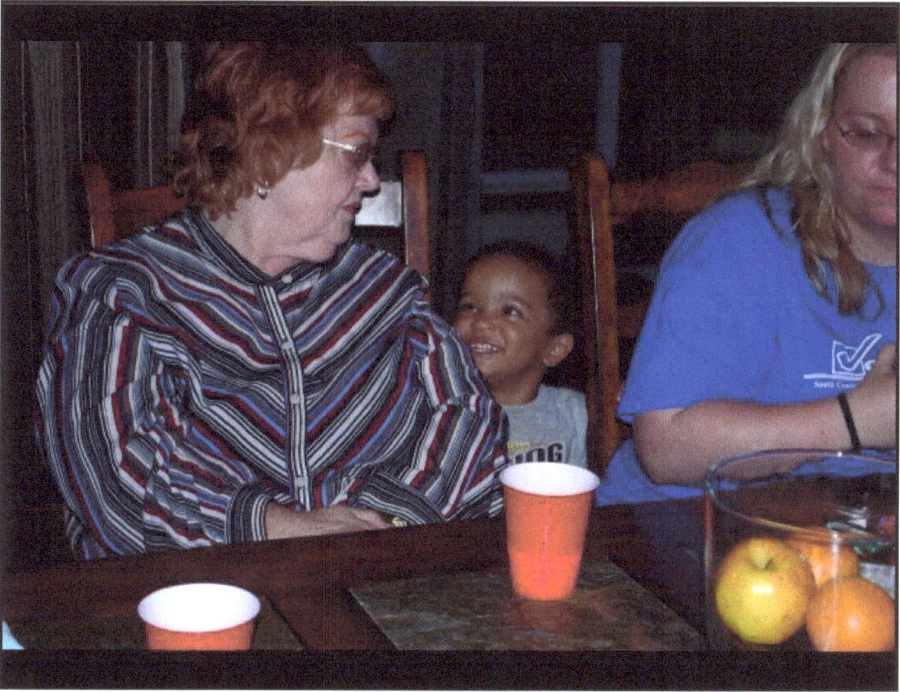

Her great-grandsons became crucial to Mom's care. She would start grinning as soon as you talked about them. When they ran through the door, they headed straight for Grammy. They loved the lift chair and would see how high it would carry them up in the air. Noah, the youngest, would climb up in her wheelchair, hold her face in his hands and give her kisses.

He loved putting lotion on her feet and making her giggle. He took such great care of her that we started calling him Dr. Noah.

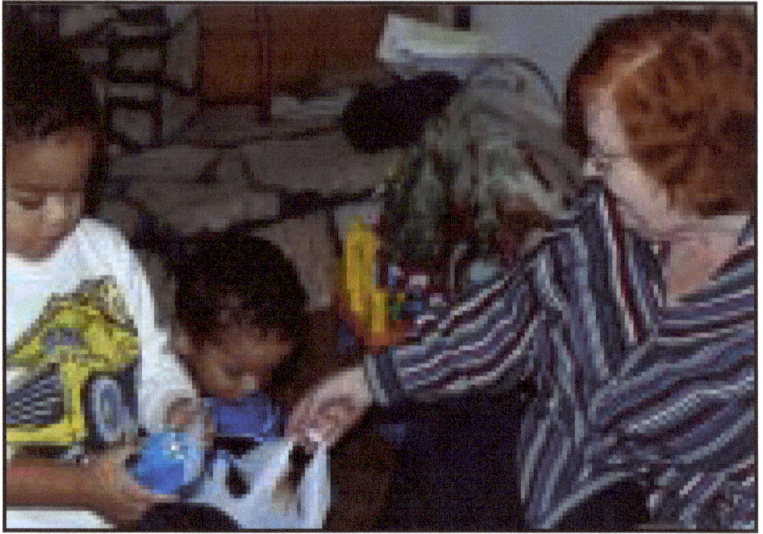

When he went to the dentist a month ago, the dentist asked what his name was. He replied, "Noah, but they call me Dr. Noah." When I had surgery last summer to remove a suspicious spot under my arm, I was not allowed to get it wet after I reopened the stitches one day. That meant I couldn't go swimming with my great-nephews for a few weeks. Noah would ask to check it. At age 3, he is still making a diagnosis if someone has a cut or bruise.

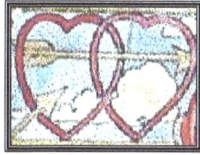

Chapter Four: The Teacher

Mom went back to school to get her teaching degree in 1972 at Emporia Kansas State Teacher's College, now called Emporia State University. The church had a student center across from the campus and Mom started taking classes. Her love for learning and for teaching never ended.

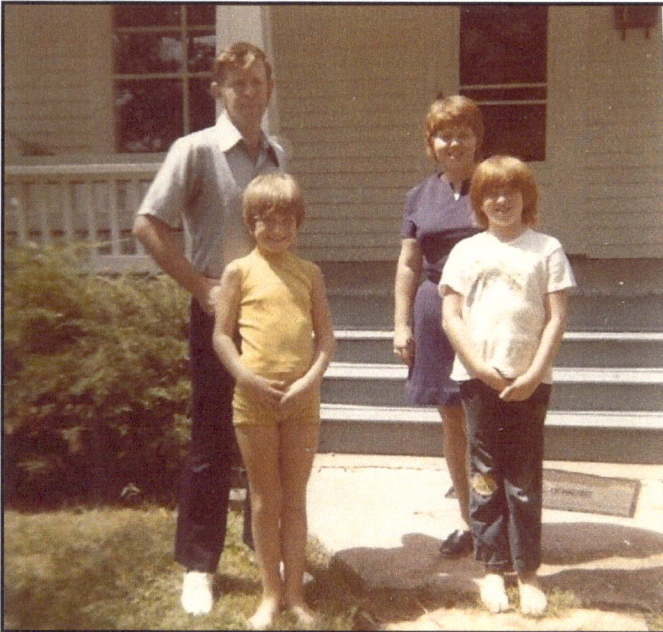

Dad, Dayna, Mom and me in front of our house
in Emporia, Kansas. (1982)

She went on to get her Master's Degree in Education at Wichita State University and her Doctor's degree in Theology from Covington Theological Seminary.

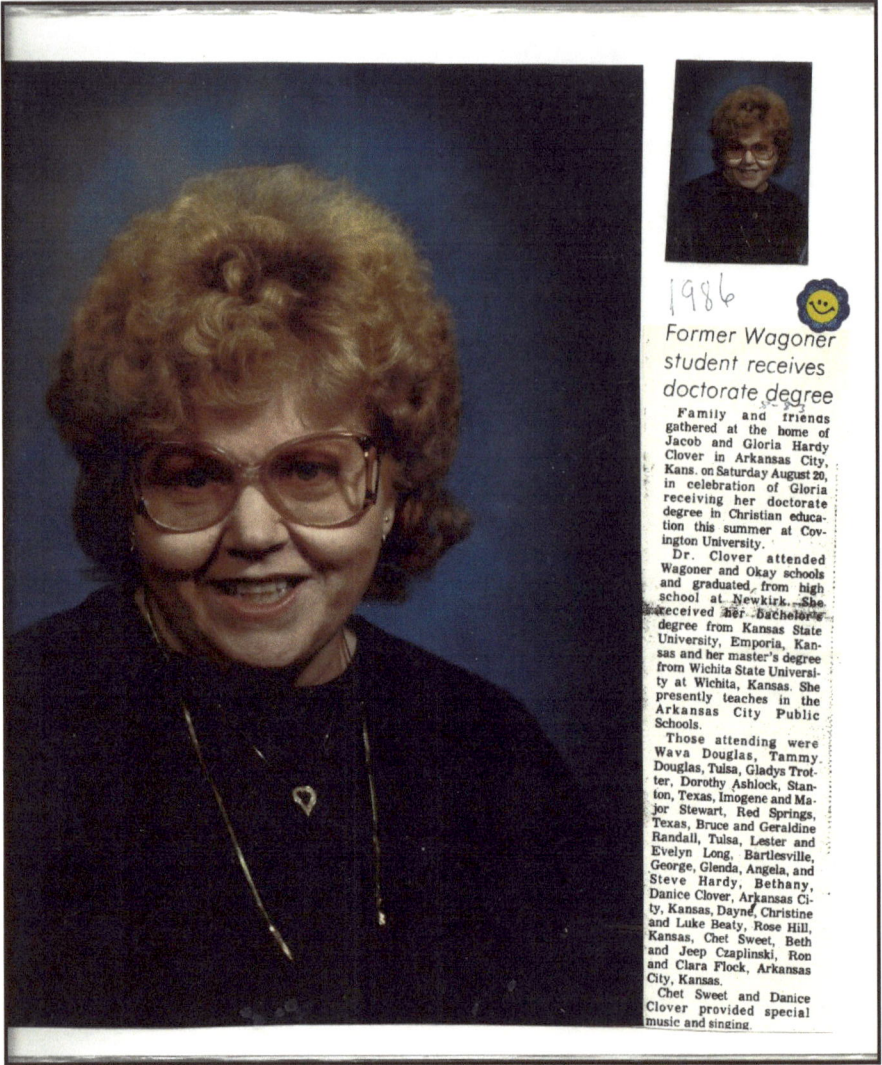

Former Wagoner student receives doctorate degree

Family and friends gathered at the home of Jacob and Gloria Hardy Clover in Arkansas City, Kans. on Saturday August 20, in celebration of Gloria receiving her doctorate degree in Christian education this summer at Covington University.

Dr. Clover attended Wagoner and Okay schools and graduated from high school at Newkirk. She received her bachelor's degree from Kansas State University, Emporia, Kansas and her master's degree from Wichita State University at Wichita, Kansas. She presently teaches in the Arkansas City Public Schools.

Those attending were Wava Douglas, Tammy Douglas, Tulsa, Gladys Trotter, Dorothy Ashlock, Stanton, Texas, Imogene and Major Stewart, Red Springs, Texas, Bruce and Geraldine Randall, Tulsa, Lester and Evelyn Long, Bartlesville, George, Glenda, Angela, and Steve Hardy, Bethany, Danice Clover, Arkansas City, Kansas, Dayne, Christine and Luke Beaty, Rose Hill, Kansas, Chet Sweet, Beth and Jeep Czaplinski, Ron and Clara Flock, Arkansas City, Kansas.

Chet Sweet and Danice Clover provided special music and singing.

I didn't know until a few years ago that her father, George Washington Hardy, could not read. She said she wanted to teach children the joy of reading, because her father never could.

She had many friends who were teachers. She loved teaching and loved students and loved the summers off. Of course, she was always taking classes, continuing her education. She had hundreds of teacher stories. One of my favorites she loved sharing occurred several years ago.

Her birthday, September 19, was always toward the start of the school year. She would tell the students she was 39. One of the last years she taught before retiring, flowers were brought in for her birthday and the students asked how old she was "39!" was Mom's reply. A quick second grader responded, "You wish!" Mom couldn't help but laugh. That student had called her bluff.

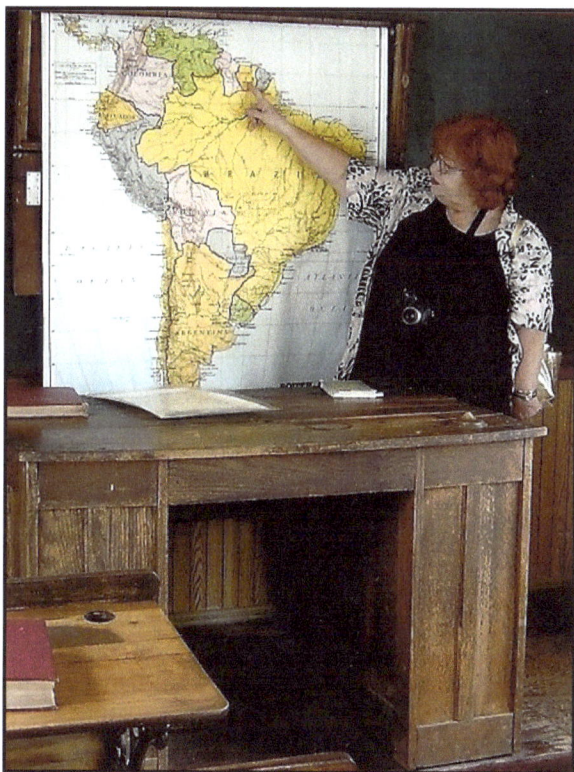
Mom at Walnut Grove, Minnesota.

Mom loved the *Little House on the Prairie* books, by Laura Ingalls-Wilder. The Little House series is based on decades-old memories of Laura Ingalls Wilder's childhood in the Midwest region of the United States during the late 19th century. (Wikipedia).

She talked about a student she had taught years ago at a country school. This student was a class clown and, after tiring of his interruptions, she finally responded, "You want to come up here and teach this class?" "Yes, I do," the fourth grader replied, and he did. Mom said he went on for about fifteen minutes and was pretty good. She made note, "Always be prepared to follow through."

She worked with hundreds of excellent teachers; one even came and played Danny Boy on the fiddle for her when she was not able to leave the house. That was always her favorite song. My name was supposed to be Danny. Guess that's how I ended up being Dan-ice, which I've had to explain every day of my life.

No, it's not *Danace*, like *Janis*; it's *Danice*, like *Denise*, except my Mom had a friend whose name was *Janice*, and she thought it should be spelled, Danice, for whatever reason. It has taught me to speak up for myself, so I forgive all of you at Home National Bank, where I have banked for 20 years, who still say, "Hello Danis."

I had the privilege of watching her teach, not only in the classroom but every day of my life. When we were small children and traveled in the car together, she would hold up an object and asked what it could be. It might have looked like a plastic lid to cottage cheese, but she would always ask, "What else could it be?" She taught us to think outside the box. The lid became a Frisbee, a plate, a hat, a saucer or even a palette. Even until the day she died I was learning from her: focus on others, always be friendly, talk *to* children, not *at* them.

I still try to instill that same creativity with my students today.

My senior year of high school I was able to spend an hour each day, helping in her classroom. She spoke to each child like he/she was a person, not just a kid. She spoke with tenderness and care, and the students loved her. Many of Mom's students have written to her and said how she was their favorite teacher. She was my favorite teacher as well.

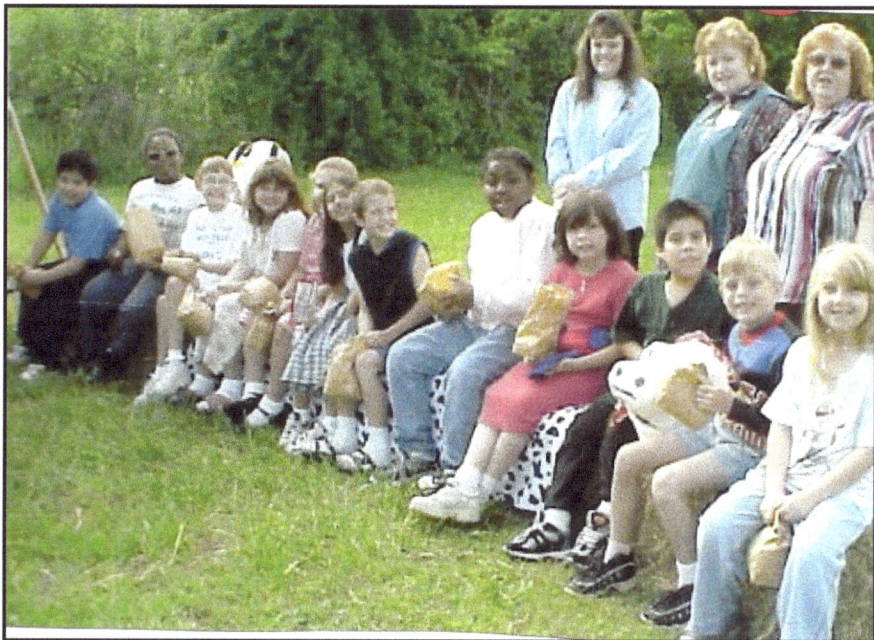

Career Day with her class,
Amy Milliman, and Aunt Evelyn as a Foster Grandparent, 2000.

Mom always said, "Where your focus goes, your energy flows." If you drive a red car, you start seeing red cars everywhere. If you focus on the positive, you start seeing the positive. If you have ALS, you start hearing about other people who have ALS. We have heard about people from all over the country, and many have heard about Mom.

Mom loved following the Iditarod Race with the Huskies in Alaska. Her second grade students loved her enthusiasm. While on a trip to Alaska a few years ago, she was thrilled when she was able to see some of the dogs that made the trip.

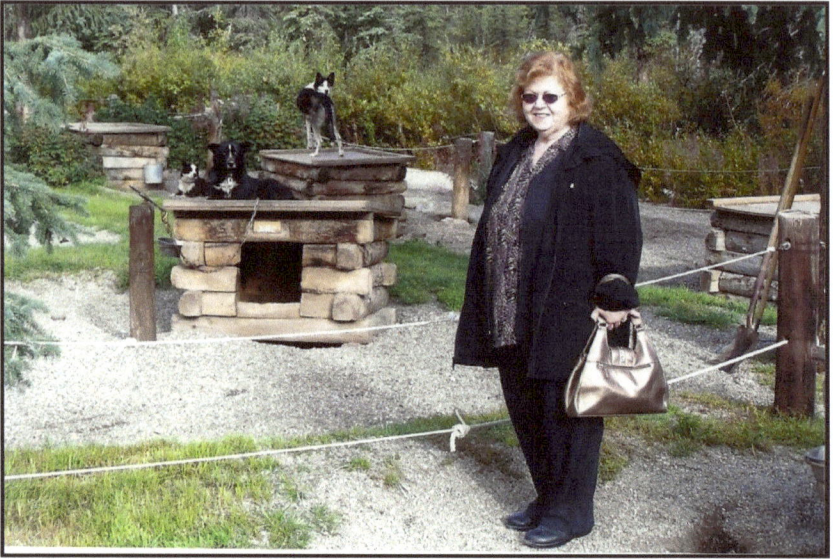

Gloria Clover in Alaska with some of the Iditarod sled dogs. (2007)

Being the youngest of ten, Mom had once thought she was adopted. Some kids were talking about it at school, and she got the notion she must have been adopted. When she came home and asked her family if she was adopted, they began laughing at the absurd thought that a family struggling to make ends meet in the little town of Wagoner, Oklahoma, would want or need to adopt another child. Mom always said she was a little disappointed at their response but grateful she was in such an amazing family

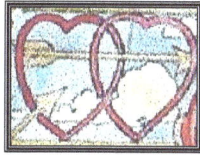

Chapter Five: A Sister

Seven wonderful ladies and two wonderful men knew my mother as a biological sister. It's taken me some time and reflection to realize how much she meant to them. Of course, I always thought of Gloria Clover as my mother. But her beautiful family thought of her as the baby. She loved that.

Her brother-in-law, Olen, always called her "little sister." She smiled every time she heard that nickname. A love for family, competition, and humor was passed down from each sibling.

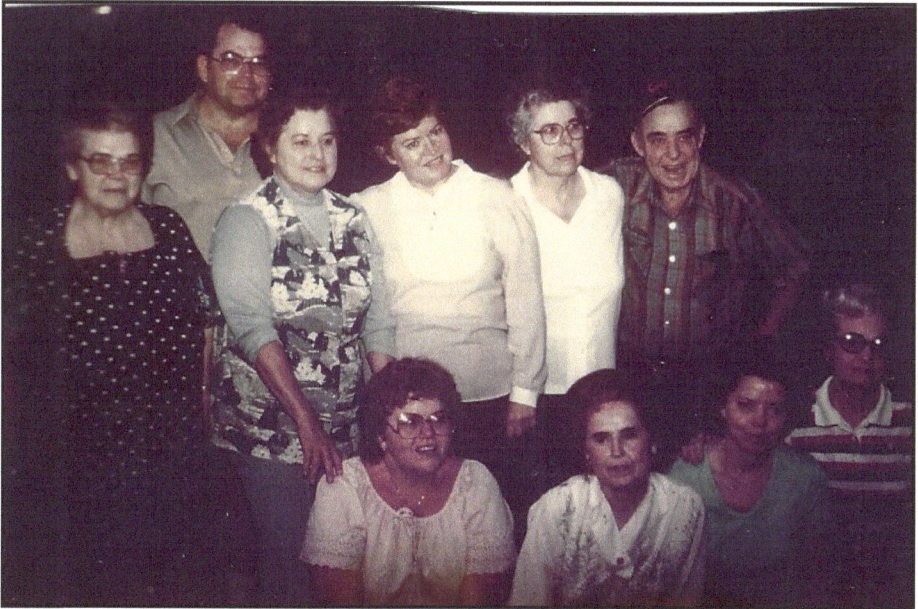

Mom with her brothers and sisters:
From left, top row: Wava, Tom, Jeannie, Evelyn, Gladys, Carl,
Bottom row: Mom,, Dorothy, Gerry and Hazel.

She would start grinning as soon as we hit the Oklahoma border when heading to a family reunion or sibling's birthday celebration. She loved being around her family, and they loved having her around.

Our famous Easter Egg hunts were always special. During our evening Scrabble games in the spring, we would start filling plastic Easter Eggs with candy and coins. I know we filled over 650 one year, but I'm sure there were more. We are still finding them in the storage room.

Mom always had a plan. Mom would take Easter eggs down to Broken Arrow, Oklahoma to cousin Tammy's house for Easter. We would all place eggs around the backyard.

She took the number of eggs and divided that by the number of people who were there and let everyone know how many eggs they could find. In the eggs, besides money and candy including (sugar-free candy for several who are diabetic) she also included notes. They were similar to a fortune cookie, except you had to do what the note said: "Sing the Star Spangled Banner," "Kiss a redhead," "Thank an aunt," "Show gratitude to a Teacher," "Say the Pledge of Allegiance," "Tell a joke."

Then by Gloria's rules, you went around the room in a somewhat orderly fashion and opened your eggs, one at a time, so everyone can see. Not unlike our Christmas traditions when we opened our stockings on Christmas Eve, oldest to youngest, there was always a plan.

April 2004 from Mom's journal entry:
We and Lyn went to Broken Arrow on the 10th; Sweet's went too, There were 33 to eat and hunt eggs. We had a groundbreaking service on the 11th Easter. M.A.G.I.C. (Most Active Group In Church) sponsored an Easter Egg Hunt with about 500 eggs.

Mom wrote in her journal about her family. Every kind word, phone call, and letter received was documented there. When a brother or sister had surgery or was hurting, she would ask us to pray. She mentioned many times how difficult it was to be the youngest of ten, believing she would out-live them all.

Then she would respond, "Do not worry about your life, what you shall eat, or what you shall drink or what you shall wear. Consider the lilies of the field. They do not labor or spin, yet not even Solomon in all his glory

28

was dressed like one of these." (Luke 12:27) She quoted scripture like an actor quoted Shakespeare. It was just part of who she was.

One of her former students stopped me on the way out of the church building last Sunday. He wanted to purchase my newest book that featured my Mom. I remembered he had been special to her. She had said he was always one of her favorites. Teachers say that have no favorites, but that wasn't true for my momma.

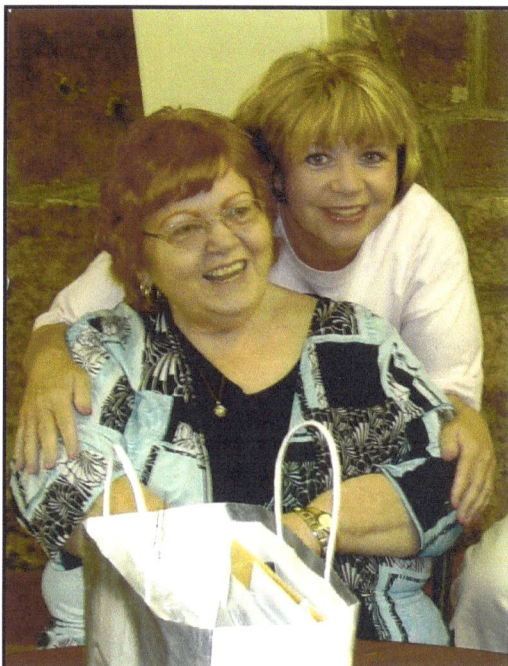

Mom and her niece, Laura Flowers at a Family Reunion.

Mom loved her nieces and nephews. She said one of her regrets was not having more children.

For some reason that surprised me. I guess being the youngest of ten, there was always a house full, and she always loved having company. She felt that being part of a large family is a very special blessing. She always received a call from all of her siblings every birthday and on many holidays.

Mom said that her mother, Grandma Hardy, always feared that the siblings would not get together after she passed. Mom often related how proud her mother and father would be that the family reunions continued to grow and that brothers, sisters and cousins still came to the stone building in Wagoner, Oklahoma to fellowship. Chet and my cousin, Stanley Ashlock and I loved to bring our guitars, mandolin, and banjo and sing old-time songs with everyone.

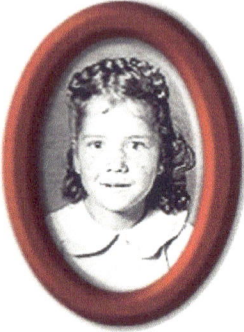

The Glory Glow

(Gloria Ann Hardy Clover)

When I first brought my date
Home-Major Stewart, a handsome,
Young Air Force captain and
We sat down in the living room,
My little red-hared, four year
Old sister, Gloria Ann, came running
And jumped into his lap.

I was horrified; then here
Came two younger sisters, Geraldine
And Evelyn and my youngest brother, George.
Major was thrilled as he did
Not have any brothers or sisters.

Gloria, or Glory as I usually call her;
Even though my father used to correct
Me as he did not like nicknames,
Looked up into Major's face and
Said "Major you come every night
Jeanne (my nickname) wants you
to come every night."

Well, Major and I soon
Married and my little sisters
And brother grew up.
Gloria became a school teacher
And worked to get her doctorate.
She has taught Arkansas City
Elementary school children for
Over twenty-five years.

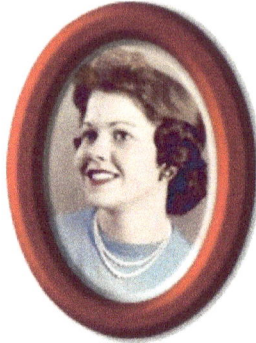

During this time her home
Has always been a place of
Warmth and welcome.
In addition to the many times
That she and her husband, Jake
And daughters, Danice and Dayna
Helped with members of their church,
Family, friends, and others.

Throughout her home is a
Collection of red-haired dolls
And often a pillow, stone
Or decoration with a four
Leaf clover design on it.

If you play a game at her
House and win you always get
A small prize and if it happens
To be Christmas Eve, everyone
There gets ten presents.
She does this because she is
The number tenth child in my family
And she wants on her tomb stone
"Here lies the true, perfect ten."

She has alway had a great
Sense of humor and years ago,
In her younger days, she showed
Her sisters a lock of her hair
And said if she ever put a rinse
On her hair, if asked, she could
Truthfully say, " This is my
Natural color."

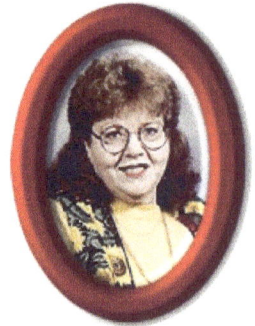

She and Jake have also helped
Dayna raise her three grandchildren
As Dayna was seriously injured
When Gloria and Jake had a car wreck
And Dayna was only six weeks old.

Shortly after her retirement,
When she had more time for
Family, friends, and grandchildren,
She was diagnosed with ALS
(Amyotropic Lateral Sclerosis).

These are only a few things
That I will relate, but if you
Ever see her smiling, loving face
You will have felt, "The Glory Glow."

Imogene Hardy Stewart
August 2008

Mom's sister, Jeannie Stewart, wrote this beautiful poem for Mom. Many people called Mom "Glo," which she enjoyed.

30

The city-wide Scrabble tournament was held at the public library. The scores were close for the top two individuals: my Mom and myself. Mom was named Scrabble Champion and has a bumper sticker that reads: Honk if you love Scrabble. I don't know if people saw the bumper sticker, or if it was her driving, but she was honked at often. I humbly claimed second place, satisfied that I had received the highest word score for the tournament. No bumper sticker, I must admit, was hard to take. You see I inherited my mother's insane competitiveness. Still, seeing that sticker on Momma's car brought a smile to my face every time.

I think I received a big, blue, soup like coffee mug with the Scrabble logo on it. Mom thought that schools should start Scrabble clubs because it helps your spelling and thinking process.

A couple of years ago I bought her the Deluxe Anniversary Scrabble board, "the kind Oprah Winfrey plays on." It was top notch, with a rotating raised board and brass trim on the racks that hold the tiles, and the tiles looked like ivory (I'm sure no elephants were harmed in the making of our Scrabble tiles). It was one of her favorite gifts of all time and did it get the use!

Mom's sister, Evelyn, came out every evening to play Scrabble, unless it was "gourmet pinochle" night. We would play Scrabble, then switch gears to play pinochle. You could set your watch to the time Evelyn arrived and the Scrabble board was placed in the center of the dining room table. I played about three nights a week with them; the competition was fierce. On a rare night I could beat them, but most of the time it was a pretty even split between my two favorite redheads as to who the winner would be. After tallying the score, Mom would announce the winner in a high, delighted voice, "It would beeeeeee... GLORIA!" I would ask her each time I won to try to say it with that same inflection. Her response was always, "I just can't do it, it doesn't sound right."

When Mom could only use sign language she would use the sign for play, wiggling her thumb and pinky, signing it was about to time to play. I will always be grateful for the game of Scrabble, and even more importantly for my Aunt Evelyn. Her journal recorded this exciting play:

June, 2005: I had a triple, triple points, went out with 2 opponents having full racks (of Scrabble Tiles).

31

As ALS continued to take its toll on my mother, she could no longer walk out to the room in which we always played Scrabble. When it became too difficult to even get the wheelchair out there, we began playing in the dining room. Later, it became impossible for her fingers to pick up the Scrabble tiles and place them on the board so she would push them forward one at a time with her index finger in the order they were to be played. My Aunt Evelyn and I would look across from each other holding back the tears, watching her lose the ability to do the one thing she loved most.

We had both played Scrabble with her long enough to know that she would, without fail, want the letters in the places that would receive the most points possible. She could see it, even if both of us could not. We would place the tiles where we thought they should go, and she would shake her head, no. Sometimes this would take considerable time, but eventually we would place the tiles in the right spot. It *always* was the one location on the board with the most points. She was the Queen of Scrabble.

On nights when I could not bear to see Mom hurting and when the wheelchair was causing her more pain than help, I would call Dad to see if Evelyn was there. He always said, "Yes." It was a relief to know Mom was doing what she loved even if the confines of ALS were making it increasingly difficult. Evelyn was an absolute saint! She was there every night, without fail, no matter how difficult it was for her, because Evelyn knew that for a few brief hours, Mom was able to use her amazing mind, and it kept her thinking about something other than her new limitations.

More than once at any given time during a game, a tear would come down Evelyn's face, then mine, then Mom's. There was an unspoken pain we all shared, knowing the time would come when we would not be able to be together again. That is, not on earth. Evelyn would reach up with a tissue and wipe Mom's mouth, as she probably did more than sixty years ago when they were children. Evelyn was the strong one. She helped keep us going when all we wanted to do was weep. She would pat Mom's hand and comfort her in every way possible.

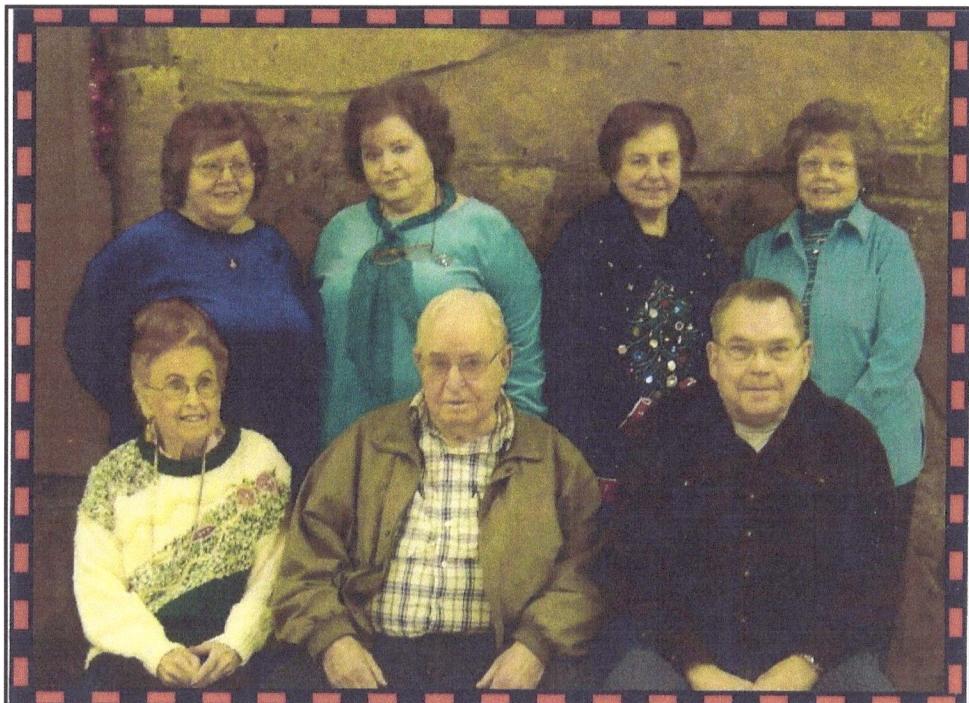

From left to Right, back row, Mom, Evelyn, Jeannie, Gerry. Front row:
Dorothy, Carl, and Tom.

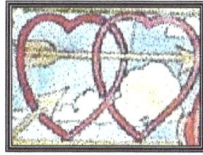

Chapter Six: Our Family

Every family gathering was filled with food and fun. Mom was the queen of organizing and creating games. She should have worked for Milton Bradley. She bought new games that would become part of each celebration. She could make the most of every puzzle, bingo, Nertz, Jjeopardy board, etc. You name it, we played it. She often made up her own rules to reward creativity. With the game Scattegories, we would get so tickled trying to create triple points with repeating the first letter such as teal tank tops, or Boston Baked Beans. The game rules state that the players get to vote whether your answers deserve all three points and Mom would often convince each player that she was worthy of the most points possible.

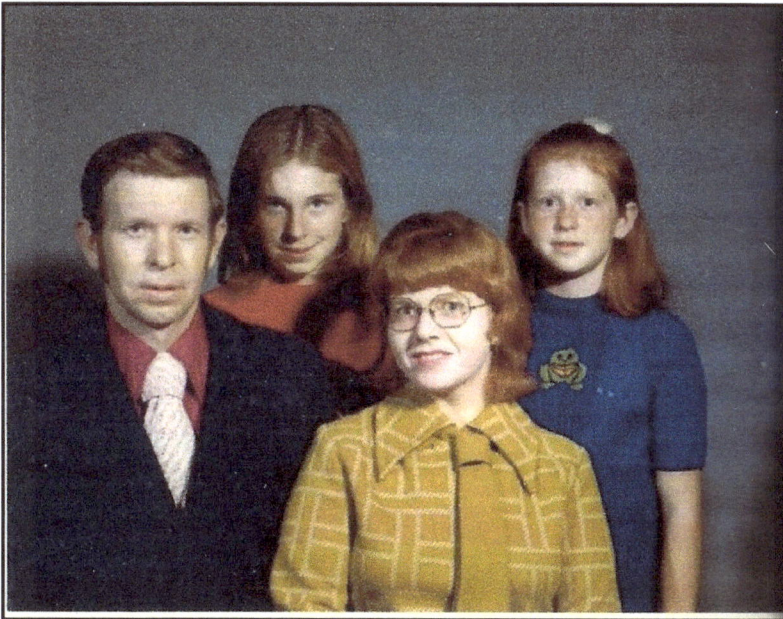

At one of our most recent birthdays when my niece, Holly and I celebrate, 1 day and 20 years apart, Mom came up with a birthday Jeopardy game. It was not unlike the well-known Jeopardy game on television with Alex Trebec as the host. She designed a board with open envelopes and headings on the top of each column, as well as point totals for each envelope. The heading topics were "Cars you've wrecked or driven," "Education," "Places you've gone," "Awards you've won," and the list went on. Ironically, our family friend, Laura Ehler, had a better memory than the rest of us and won my birthday Jeopardy game. Of course, there were prizes. Mom was known for giving out prizes for everything. Whether it was a knick knack, a plastic hanger, or a piece of chocolate, you always won something.

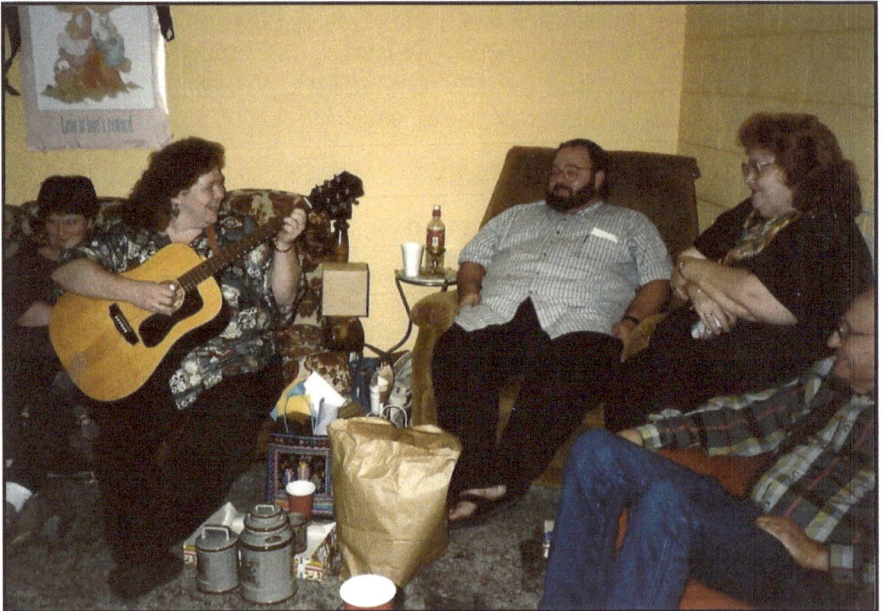

Dayna, Danice, Chet, Mom and Uncle Olen
on Chet's 40th Birthday Surprise Party

When I left for college, Mom and I both cried. Every time I came home from college and had to leave again for Oklahoma Christian College, we cried. We both missed each other so much.

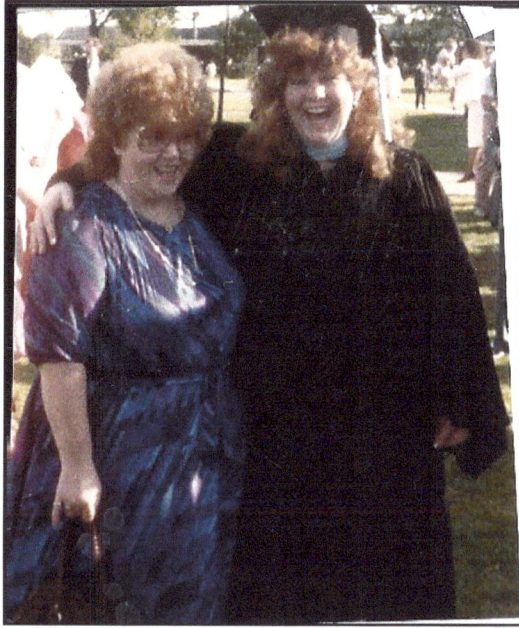

Graduating from Oklahoma Christian College,
Magna Cum Laude, 1986.

Mom and Dad always had people over for fellowship. That's what we called inviting friends to Bible Studies, cards, volleyball, or Soul Talks. Mom created a Bible study lesson plan. She felt that Bible studies should be just that: studies about the Bible, not just one man spouting what he knows about God's word, but everyone in the Word of God, studying, reading and sharing. She created a format called Soul Talks with questions and study guides. She understood that many people learn best by discussion.

Our home was filled with missionaries visiting from other countries, music groups that needed a place to stay and people who were struggling and needed a safe place for a while. Consequently our vacations were trips to Wisconsin for a door knocking campaign to help with Vacation Bible School. We also went to Williamstown Bible College where I first heard Keith Lancaster's group *His Image* which soon became *Acappella*. I believed if I learned every part of every song, I just might get to sing for the Lord someday. I am so grateful that God blessed Chet and me with that opportunity.

Of course things had changed at home. My sister had divorced and moved back in with Mom and Dad with her three children.

My sister's three children are Chrissy, Dale and Holly. We love them with all we've got: heart, mind and spirit. We all took part in helping Dayna raise them.

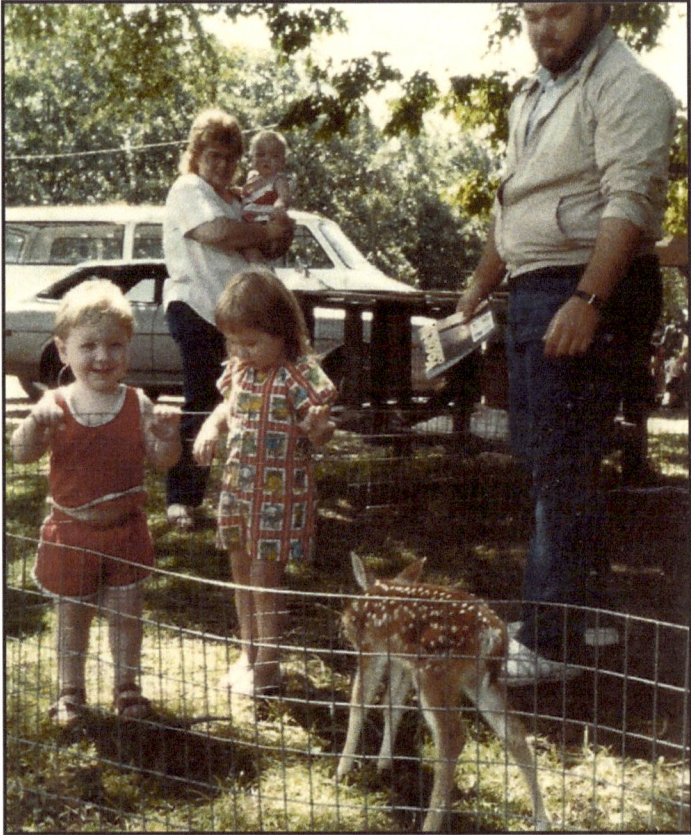

Lucas Dale, Mom and Holly, Christine and Chet, 1986

Holly had two boys, Gabe and Noah.

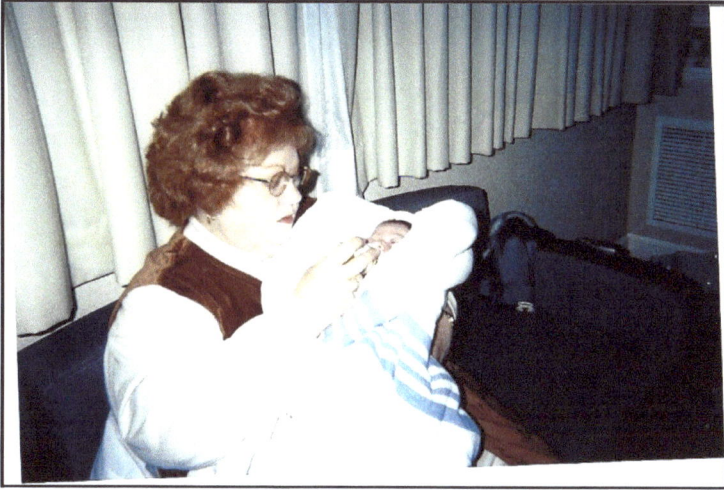

Mom with Gabriel Harper, Durant, Oklahoma. 2004

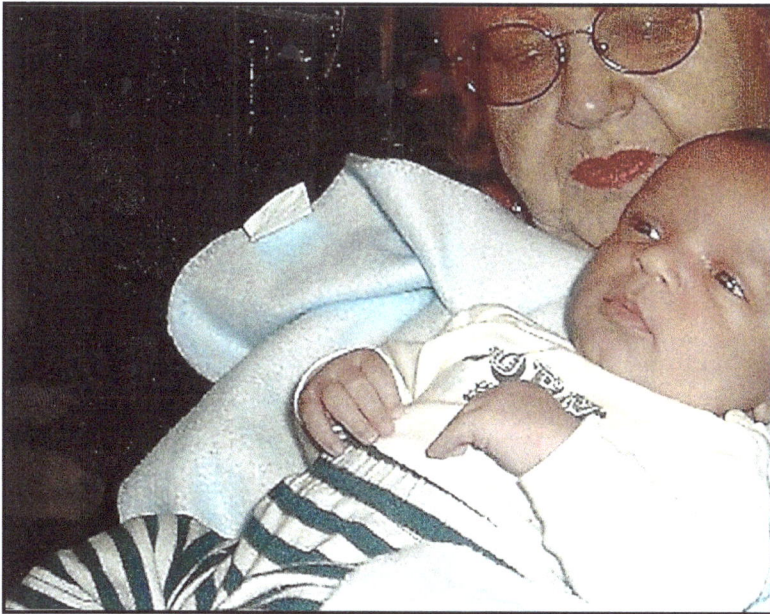

Mom with Noah Harper, 2006

Gloria became the most involved, most loving, affectionate, great-grandma you could ever meet. Her friends at McDonald's saved the cards that came with their gift certificates so she could plug the numbers on the back into the computer for a college fund called U Promise…at the huge amount of fifteen cents per card number. It started slowly but certainly added up. She wanted to be sure her great-grandchildren had the chance of an education. One day going through McDonalds' drive-thru, I used some gift certificates I had received. The clerk asked if she could keep the back of the gift certificates for a friend.

I said, "Well, I'm sorry, but I'm saving them for my great-nephews."

She replied, "That's okay; Gloria gets plenty."

"Gloria who?" I responded.

"Gloria Clover, one of our best customers!" she answered.

"That's my mother!" I grinned back.

"They're going to the same place, then," she giggled.

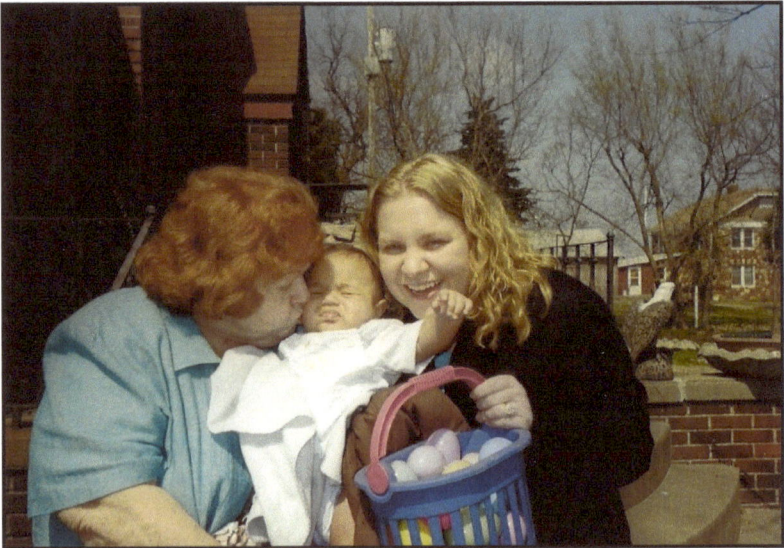

Mom, Gabe & Holly on his first Easter Egg Hunt.

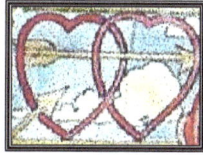

Chapter Seven: Mama's Family

The Hardy bunch is an amazing, close knit, prayerful, loving, giving, supportive group of brothers and sisters. Nothing delighted me more at family reunions than to sit and listen to them retell stories about growing up together. Everyone has a different slant on each story. Mom, being the youngest, had the view from the floorboards of the car, going all the way from Oklahoma to California.

Her sisters tell a different tale. Since Mom was the baby of the family, the siblings insisted that their parents were worn out by the time she came along. Nevertheless, my cheeks would hurt from grinning while they all chimed in on their particular memory. Mom wrote a book several years back and asked me to illustrate it. It was entitled, *When Gladys Came Home*. There's a children's book called *The Relatives Came*, (Rylant, 1993), and Mom loved reading it to her second grade classes because it reminded her of her own childhood.

She would say, "Monday was laundry day, we always had beans." I never made the connection, until I got older and realized you could put a pot of beans on for a long time and focus on chores, so that's why Monday was laundry *and* bean day.

My Aunt Evelyn was out at Mom and Dad's one evening to play Scrabble, and I realized I had put my shirt on inside out. Evelyn said, "Our momma would say, 'That'll never be noticed on a galloping horse.'" I think I relate to that one. Sometimes we go through life worrying about the little things. Mom would always quote the scripture, "Who of you, by worrying, can add a single hour to your life." (Matthew 6:27)

My Aunt Wava was saying one day, "If I was younger I'd set my cap for Charlie Pride."

My grandpa responded, "Lord, have mercy on old age."

41

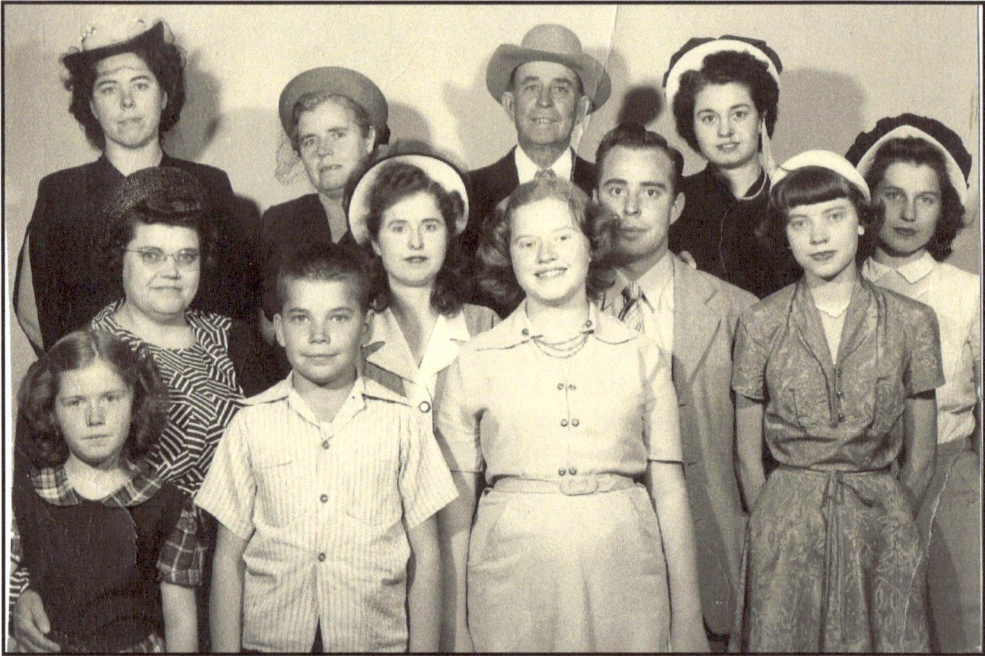

From top left: Gladys, Grandma Hardy, Grandpa Hardy, Hazel,
Second row: Wava, Dorothy, Carl, Jeannie,
Bottom row: Gloria, Tom, Evelyn and Gerry.

Mom loved retelling the story of when her older sister Gladys came back to Oklahoma from California to visit. She always brought homemade jam. Mom thought it was strange that the family gave Gladys homemade jam to take home, when that is what she brought to them all the way from California. Gladys would say as they were packing up to leave, "Why don't ya'll come home with us?" Mom could not understand why they couldn't all go.

My cousin, Gary Ashlock said that when they came to Wagoner from Texas for Christmas, they knew there wouldn't be gifts because things were tough. However, they also knew that Mom, who was closer to their age than to his mother, Mom's sister Dorothy, would have a gift for all three boys. She would go to the second hand store in town and spend her own money to get "funny books" so they would have something to open on Christmas. I never knew that until last week. She was a giver even as a teenager, always thinking of others.

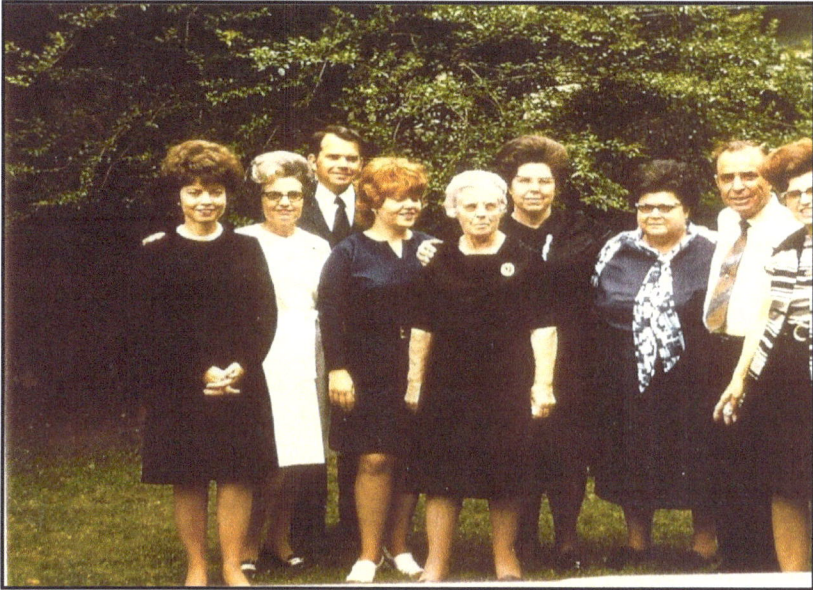

Gerry, Hazel, Tom, Mom, Grandma Hardy, Gladys, Wava, Carl and
Dorothy at Grandpa Hardy's funeral.

It's taken me some time to appreciate how difficult ALS has been on
Mom's siblings. I guess I was preoccupied, thinking of how it was affecting
Mom, Dad, my sister, my nieces, my nephew, great-nephews and myself.
My cousin called one night to check on me to see how I was holding up.
She said one of Mom's sisters had not stopped crying. Then I stopped and
imagined what I would feel like if my sister was given the same diagnosis. I
don't know what I'd do. For now, I write.

I miss my Mom. I miss her laugh, her sense of humor, her ideas
and her willingness to go anywhere, and be up for any adventure. Several
years ago there was a little golf course on the edge of town. It was a Par
Three Course, so the holes were short and renting a golf cart was cheap.
We'd take the grandkids and a friend or two and go out and play a round of
nine holes. She always said her sister Hazel could have gone pro. Hazel
had taught her how to hold the putter parallel to the hole. Mom always
played with style, no matter the game. She was never a sore loser, but she
DID like to win! She was competitive, yes, always giving it her all.

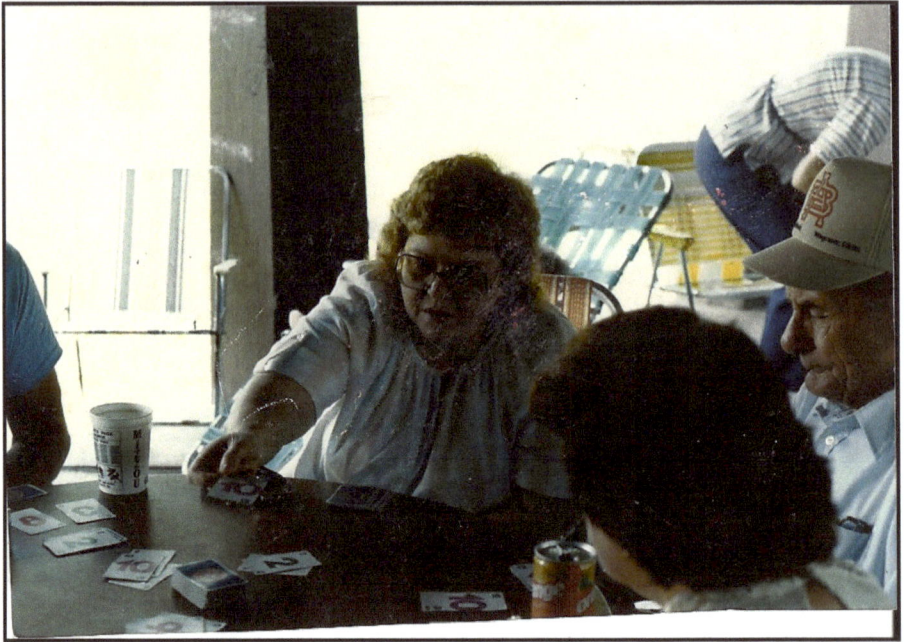

Gloria playing cards at the Hardy Family Reunion.

I ran to the Chinese restaurant in town last night to pick up supper. The owner asked me how Dad was. I replied that he was doing fine.

She said, "I miss your mother."

I was surprised.

She said, "My mother died five years ago. Your mother asked why we close, and I told her my mom die. She send me flowers. No customer ever do that before."

I simply responded, "That sounds like her."

She always had an ongoing bill at the local flower shop. I'll never know all the people she sent flowers to, or all the good she did.

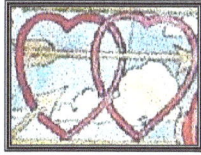

Chapter Eight: Dad

Dad can fix anything: cars, busses, RV's, plumbing, electrical, construction, leaky swimming pools. You name it. He's a "Jake of all Trades." In fact, that's what he called himself after he retired the first time. He had a handyman business where he worked for people doing odd jobs. He was always there for us, between working as a government meat inspector to working at Total Petroleum to preaching at little towns when they needed someone.

Dad was always building things for us. We had the most amazing doll house on wheels with carpet and tile on the floors inside. As my sister and I grew up, he made playhouses for us to pretend in. When we moved from Emporia, we brought our play house with us and put stuffed animals in it and called it Clover's Ark. Dad had an old wooden boat that he put the playhouse on and added a Rambler dashboard so we could act like Noah and steer the ship, we had captain's hats and everything. Dad could repair anything, create amazing things, and fix whatever was broken. But he could not fix ALS. None of us have that chromosome that asks for help. This situation was no exception.

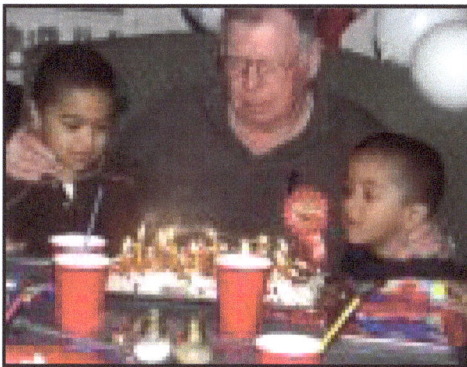

Dad's birthday with Gabe and Noah
helping to blow out the candles.

None of us ever went into nursing. It just wasn't our calling. I must say before I go on, that I have the utmost respect for anyone in the medical field, who dedicates their life to helping others at such difficult times.

My dad became the most amazing caregiver I have ever seen. He would not leave my mother's side. He slept in a recliner for months when she could not sleep in a bed. When a hospital bed was brought in, he moved his recliner closer to the bed so he could be there whenever she needed anything. He installed a cordless doorbell that she could push if he was doing laundry in the basement or in the other room mixing her vitamins for the feeding tube. He kept a list on a clipboard on the wall in the kitchen, in case something should happen to him, so that we would know what to do to help Mom. It told us what medications she needed, what time they were given, how they were given, what protein or juices she could handle and how to reach him.

The two times he was not there, she fell. Dad went to Oklahoma City to help my sister, whose husband had a very difficult time after heart surgery. I convinced Dad that I could handle anything that came up, but I was wrong. I didn't know that Mom's legs were no longer dependable. I don't think she knew either.

When I tried to help her move from the wheelchair to her lift chair, we both went down. I got her to the ground safely, but no matter how we tried I could not get her back up. I called for help as she began to cry silently. She couldn't make a sound so all you could see was her mouth open and the tears coming down her face.

That, in turn, always made me cry as well. Help arrived in the way of my husband, my nephew, his wife, my niece, and her husband, and we were both relieved.

When Dad made it home, and heard about the fall, he shook his head and started crying.

"I knew I shouldn't have gone. I told you I never should have left. This would never have happened." We both cried.

I've never seen one man work so hard to care for one woman. He did laundry, dishes, maintained her medicine, communicated with nurses, translated what Mom wanted or needed, paid bills, kept the house, and even put on her makeup for her.

He had the most difficulty with accepting help. That's the "Clover Way." My dad's dad was the same way. If he couldn't take care of it, he would kill himself trying to.

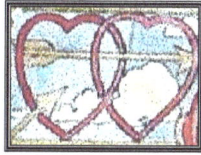

Chapter Nine: Her Friends

One of Mom's best friends gave her a sign she kept on the wall, which reads, "It's Great to Have Friends to Grow Old With, You Go First." Mom always said, "Have friends who are older than you and younger than you, and you will never be lonely."

She had friends of all ages. She had her McDonald's buddies: the group of folks from the community who meet at the local McDonald's in Ark. City.

For years they would watch the traffic, discuss the weather and keep up with each others' families. They celebrated birthdays and anniversaries and checked in on each other. Mom even organized contests at McDonald's. They would place nickel bets on how tall certain customers were. Someone would eventually go up and ask the customer how tall they were, and the one closest to the right height would receive all the nickels.

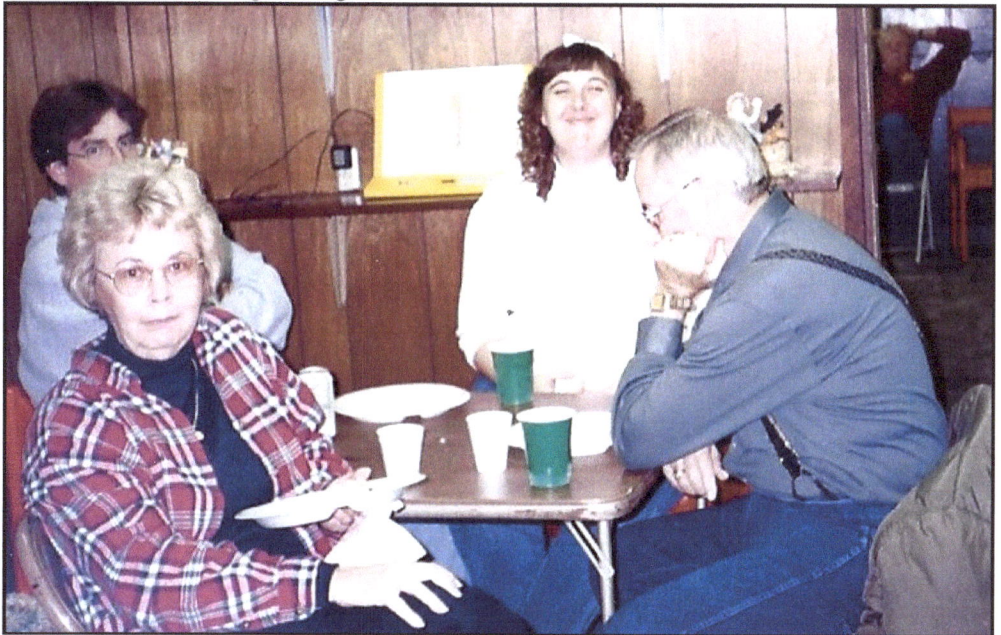

Jim McNulty, Clara Flock, Debbie McNulty and Ron Flock
at Mom and Dad's.

She had church friends who wee faithful to pray and visit and try to understand why this was happening to "Glo." The cards she received were kept in a huge basket. I still have them. I read them when I'm feeling low and start fearing that she is forgotten. Her church friends brought food and friendship.

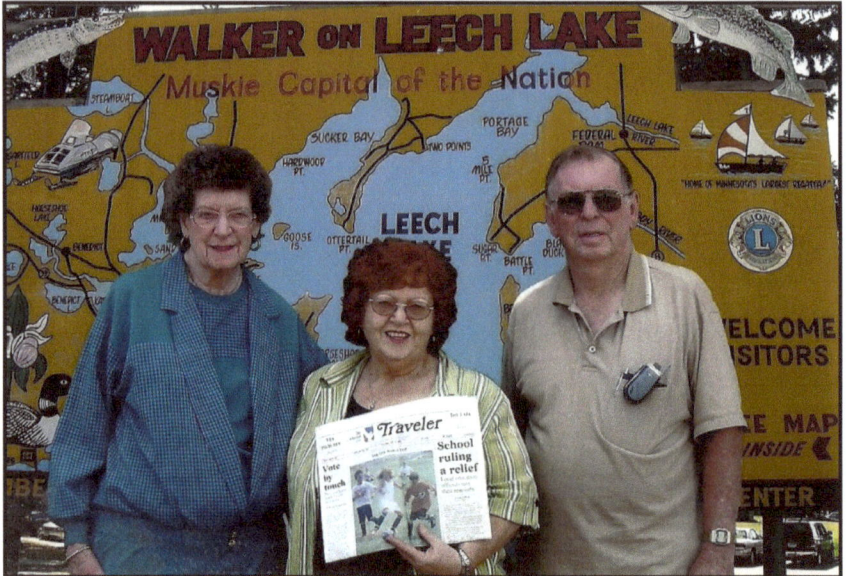

Jeri Frambers, Mom and Dad in Walker, Minnesota 2006.

One of Mom's dearest friends were Howard and Jeri Frambers. They were church, pinochle and McDonald's friends. Our singing group Revival was heading to Louisiana for a few concerts when Howard was very ill. Mom asked us to go by their house on Eighth Street and sing Howard a song before we left. I looked in his eyes and knew it would be the last time I saw him here on earth, and it was. Mom and Dad remained great friends with Jeri and spent some time together almost everyday. I think Mom thought of her like a sister. One afternoon Jeri did not make it to McDonald's. Mom tried to call her and she didn't answer the phone. Mom was certain something was wrong and insisted they go by her house. She didn't answer the door, but her car was in the carport. They finally got in the house and found that Jeri had a stroke. We arrived at the same time the ambulance did. Jeri spent time in a rehabilitation hospital in Wichita and Mom went to see her often. She wanted to take care of her, but her son insisted on moving her closer to his home in Minnesota. Mom and Dad made the trip to see her.

Hewins, Kansas probably isn't on the map, unless they do one of those close ups when a tornado is coming and you hear of towns you never heard of your whole life. We enjoyed some wonderful times at Hewins. Our family friends, Don and Norma Cole, have some land over there, and we celebrated almost every possible holiday you could at the camp out there. Mom even kept a Hewins photo album of all the good times shared.

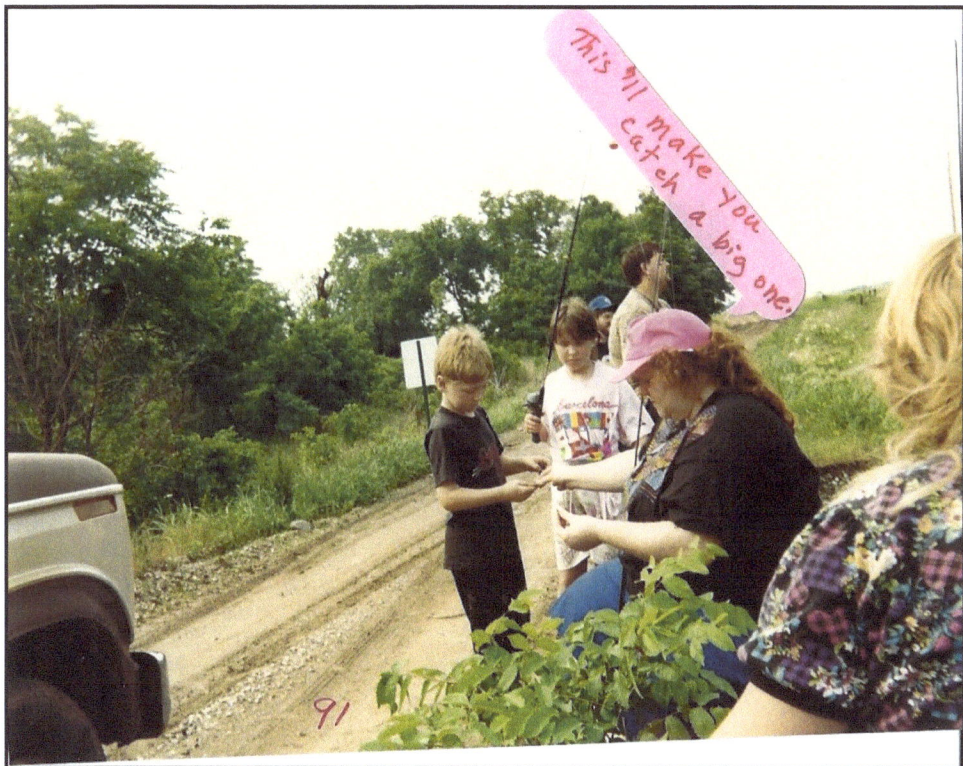

Lucas Dale, Chrissy, Jim McNulty, Brian Cole, Danice
and Holly fishing at Hewins.

We would fish during the day, catch sun perch for bait, and then the men and boys would set lines for catfish at night. There was a time when we all had campers, truck toppers and tents set up there year round.

One night, while Chet and I were sleeping in our camper that fit over a truck,(mind you, minus the truck), we were awakened in the pitch dark by falling five feet to the ground when the topper bed we were sleeping in had rotted out. Down we went. Waking up so abruptly in the dark at a campsite by the river, I yelled, "I'm stepping on glass! I'm stepping on glass!" My husband Chet calmly replied, "Get up! Those are sticks, we are now outside!"

When Dayna's kids were little, it was a great place to get away because it only costs you and the flat tires you get from trying to go down a road made of huge rocks. We started out taking the usual hotdogs, hamburgers and chips but then, as Mom would have it, we coordinated Stir fry nights, Mexican fiestas and bar-be-cue.

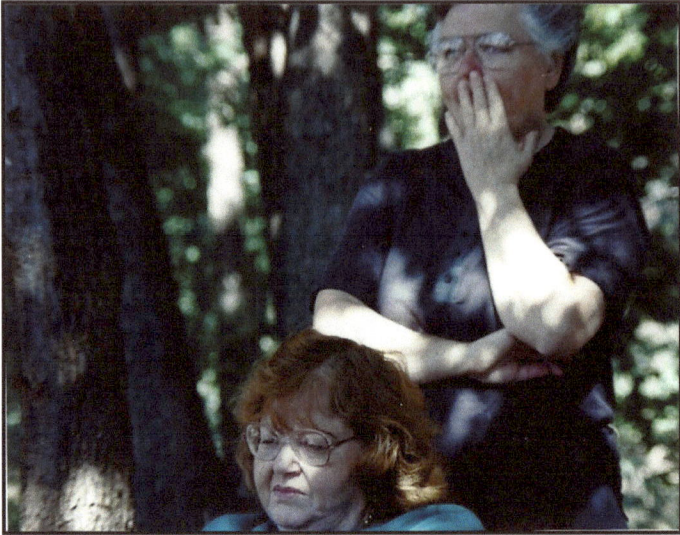

Mom and Norma Cole at the farm in Hewins, Kansas

Playing cards, fighting flies and mosquitoes, playing dominoes, singing with our guitars and shooting off fireworks were some of the main activities at Hewins. Running after fireworks on a four-wheeler with a bucket of water was a regular occurrence when the season was dry. Watching Chet wrestle a five foot long black snake back up the hill after it decided to surprise Norma's granddaughter while she was on the swing. You've never seen a group of campers move so quickly to get out of the way of a snake.

Swimming in the Caney River, bathing at Ozro in our swimsuits, sharing a bar of soap, so long as it floated, were some good times. Worshipping at the Hewins Church of Christ, the oldest in the state of Kansas, with two light bulbs hanging from the ceiling and outhouses for bathrooms. We learned about God's word and sang every verse of every slow hymn you've never heard. I can't help but smile thinking of those days. Good times.

We would all walk in, hoping we weren't bringing too much mud from camping, and someone would say, "Hey, the good singers are here!" Mom would smile proudly, and take all the credit she could carry, just grateful to be grouped in with the "good singers." Ironically, we weren't able to make it one holiday, and when Dad and Mom came in, someone again commented on how good the singing would be, and Mom knew they were in trouble. Mom said that folks kept turning around to see what happened or what was missing, and she could only turn red. Not only was the singing not good, but it truly was a "joyful noise unto the Lord." (Psalms 89:4) And that's all that truly matters.

She had pinochle friends: couples and ladies she played cards with for over twenty years. Well, I've been playing with them for twenty years, so it must be at least thirty years. The ladies group has renamed themselves the Gloria Clover Pinochle group. They still gather each month to fellowship and play cards. It's hard to play now without Mom. She insists in her last letter to me, "Keep on playing pinochle with the ladies. They are good women and will always be there for you."

She had this wonderful habit of bidding more quietly than usual, if she didn't have a very good hand. I called it her Meryl Streep bid. She should have been an actress. Consequently, when some of the players started losing some of their hearing, she would still sort of whisper the bid, hoping they got the hint to bid over her. It was a scene from a situation comedy when they start asking, "Gloria, did you bid?" and she would whisper back, "fifty-three," and they replied, "Whad'ya say?" And she would have to just come out and say it. The whole table, except of course, her pinochle partner, knew what she was doing.

Mom also had swimming pool friends. In our home I grew up in on Fourth Street, we put in a swimming pool in the backyard. We liked it so much, Dad and I dug a huge hole, and after 15 truckloads of dirt were taken out, while we listened to the Oak Ridge Boys eight track tape of Ya'll Come Back Saloon, we put the pool in the ground. We liked that so much. Dad, who could build anything, put up field stone walls between the house and the garage and we swam all year around. We put a volleyball net across the round pool and started playing water volleyball. We would have up to thirty ladies in that pool. You'd be surprised how hard church ladies can spike a volleyball when the water is only four feet deep. We had some great times out there.

Dayna's kids were swimming when they were toddlers. It was great, clean exercise, and something we all enjoyed. Eventually Dad filled in the pool and turned the whole room into a game room, but I'll never forget how much fun we had.

Mom was always very conscientious about exercise. We played volleyball with a homemade court beside the house. She was always walking, getting her 10,000 steps in. She was always finding money when she walked. We joked that since she was barely five feet tall, she was closer to the ground.

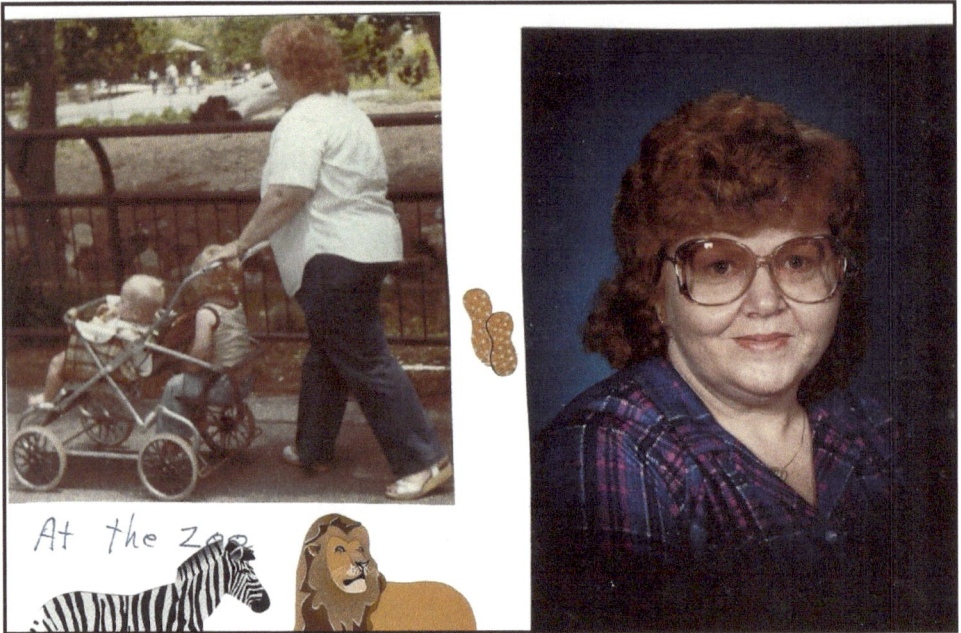

Here she is with Holly and Dale at the Sedgwick County Zoo, Wichita, Kansas in 1985.

She got an elliptical machine and a treadmill and loved to read magazines while she walked on the treadmill. She was a speed reader and consumed books and magazines as fast as she received them. She only read non-fiction, and did not understand why anyone would waste time reading anything that wasn't true. She would donate her Christian books to preachers and friends and made huge book donations to church libraries. She would always rate the book from a 1 to a 10, and if it was above an 8 she would re-read it. So if you stumble on a book with a number and date in the front cover, it may have been one of hers.

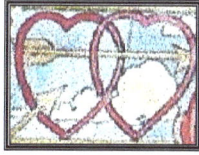

Chapter Ten: The Encourager

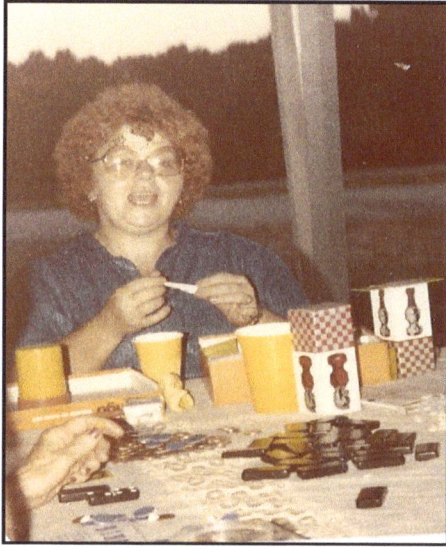

Calling Bingo at the 1980 Reunion

Some people struggle to find their gifts. Not their presents for a birthday or Christmas, but their gifts, their talents, their God-given guided area of expertise. Mom had many gifts. But the one that shined the brightest is her gift of encouragement.

I've asked our friends to share some things they remember about how Gloria encouraged them:

Evelyn Shoup wrote: "Gloria loved books and sharing them with her friends. When I browse through my books, I find so many with a personal note written inside - "To Evelyn, from Glo." I have many things that she gave me through the years - books, folders about Frances Willard, and other very effective and creative teaching ideas. I was searching today for some materials for a teacher, and ran across one of the books she gave me. Not a day goes by that I don't think about her."

55

Kay Glover wrote: "I was truly blessed when Danice and Chet joined our families. Gloria has filled me with wonderful memories. The games at holidays are among the best. Gloria had this look like 'so you think you're winning because I want you too,' then the smile got bigger and the eyes got brighter, and you found that she was winning!! Gloria was one of the most giving and thankful people I have ever known, not one day goes by that I don't think of her. On my dresser is the doll from Gloria next to a rabbit from my Mom. I love seeing them every day. They make me smile. I think that was the plan. Gloria gave gifts of life and living to every person she met."

Steve Martin wrote: "She told Carol and me that we should go ahead and have more children if we wanted. She said our kids (she had both girls in class) were well parented, and we doing a great job. That was very sweet of her to say and encouraging to us. Our girls loved Mrs. Clover! It didn't convince us to have any more though....."

Dallas Jordan shares, "I remember when I first met Gloria. She made me immediately feel that I was, (and somehow, had always been), a welcome and valued member of what I now know is a uniquely special big circle of loved ones. She made me wish I was, and strive to be, a better person. There are usually very few people in our lives that openly and sincerely represent the loving grace of God. Gloria is high on that list for an awful lot of people. People that are fortunate and forever linked together for having known her."

Loretta Vann, "I loved Gloria. She was such an encourager and always made me feel like I could do more than I felt like I could. What a blessing to have known her."

"She was a wonderful woman and an amazing teacher. She had a great impact on Emily and has always been one of her favorites," Kathy Kendrick.

"Mrs. Clover was one of my favorite teachers," David Barclay, Jr, Omaha, Nebraska.

"Mrs. Clover was a wonderful teacher and will be missed," Jeff Faber, Oklahoma, City.

"Mrs. Clover was my all-time favorite teacher! She and I had lunch together at Long John Silvers as a special reward for reading the most books in my class. I will never forget her and owe my career as a writer to her persistence to get me published in the Gumball Gazette."
Charissa Struble, Orlando, Florida.

Bruce Randall, Mom's nephew from Tulsa, Oklahoma was asked to speak at Mom's Celebration of Life Service. Bick, as we all called him, was born on Mom's birthday, September 19, and Mom loved him dearly. Bruce shared, "...she found worth in people, not things...she kept a sense of wonder that she never lost...she had the most ultimate confidence in the providence of God that, even if she was struck with ALS, it was for a purpose. That purpose was to praise Him and that she did."

"Danice, your mother touched many lives in our community. She had a loving, caring family that was there for her in deeds and with many prayers. Someone said, 'to have any lasting impact on the world, we must focus our energy on people, not profits or success. If we can help one person, our efforts will never be in vain.' Know that God never makes a mistake." Maredith Watson, Arkansas City, Kansas
.

"I will always think of Aunt Gloria with fond memories and will miss her soft chuckle, quick wit, and uncanny game playing skills." Edwina Alexander, California.

"I will always equate Scrabble with Aunt Gloria. And where did she ever get those dice shaped like tiny little pigs? Aunt Gloria could find the most unusual games. A visit with Aunt Gloria meant fun and laughter," Terri Cochran, Louisiana.

"Words will never be enough to express how very much Aunt Gloria meant to me. Family gatherings will never be the same without her, the games, prizes and incredible thoughtfulness for others. She added years to Mom's life by paying Mom's way to Weight Watchers so many years ago. I would have never gone to Garnett and met Mike without Aunt Gloria's influence!!! My initial "professional wear" upon graduating from college was bought on "credit" at "Mode O'Day" in Ark City. She was and is such an angel." Mike and Tammy DeVault, Tulsa, OK.

"I know that you will miss her as much as I had over the last few months of not waiting on her. She always had a smile on her face when she came into the Sirloin Stockade and could always make me smile even when I was having a bad day." Judy Secrest, from Kansas.

Terry Cheatham from Tennessee said, "she just always made me feel like the greatest singer in the world. Her comments on songs that I sang make me feel good to this day! She always liked the song you wrote for me that I sang, "My Prayer." What a tremendous woman and Christian lady!!"

Cheryl Bolack, "When I first came to Ark City to teach 37 years ago, Gloria was one of the first teachers that made me feel welcome at IXL. She was an awesome teacher who thoroughly enjoyed sharing books and stories with her students. I would go in to get a student, and Gloria would be reading. I couldn't leave because I wanted to listen to the story, too."

Bret Testerman from Florida, "Jake and Gloria have been a part of my life for as long as I can remember. Some of my fondest memories, as a child, was my sister Jaime and I spending time with Dayna and Danice over at the Clover home. Gloria was always such a constant source of love and joy. Now looking back, at age 45, I realize that God used Jake and Gloria to help in building a foundation for faith that has sustained me into adulthood and has now been passed on to my own children. During all the years that Danice and I sang together in college, Gloria was such a wonderful source of encouragement. My life was greatly enriched by knowing Gloria Clover."

Judith Admire: "I will always remember her kindness, courtesy and charity toward others. Gloria was a real lady, and it was a delight to work with her. Even after all the time that has passed, the impact you made on our lives is strong. Rob sends his love to his favorite art teacher. You have your mother's gift, and we hope it will be a blessing to you and to others."

My mother encouraged me every day of my life. When I wanted to play an instrument she said, "Now you can pick anything you want to play, but a guitar you can carry with you, a piano is harder to move." So I began to play the guitar in fifth grade.

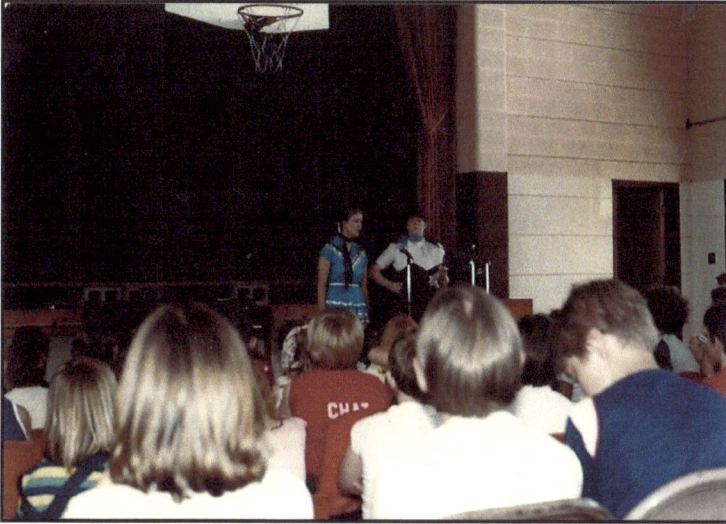

Donja Hayes Cary and Danice Clover Sweet
singing at 1950's Day at IXL School. (1983)

When our town held a local talent show, Mom insisted my friend, Donja Hayes (Cary), and I enter the contest and sing Blowin' In The Wind. I thought I'd learned the chord,s and we thought we knew the song, but that little stage at Spark's Music Store on Summit Street in downtown Arkansas City, Kansas scared the words and chords right out of us. I knew we would never sing in front of anyone again. Next card party Mom and Dad had, Mom suggested we get up and try singing again.

My friend Debbie Cole (McNulty) and I went to see the movie, The Buddy Holly Story. I came home so inspired that Debbie and I put together a Buddy Holly Medley. I figured out the chords to the guitar, and we started singing. Old favorites like, "If You Knew Peggy Sue," "That'll Be The Day" and "It's So Easy To Fall In Love" became our little concert tunes. Any couples that came over to play pitch or pinochle became our audience. Mom would say,

"You go get your guitar and practice and come down and sing for us."

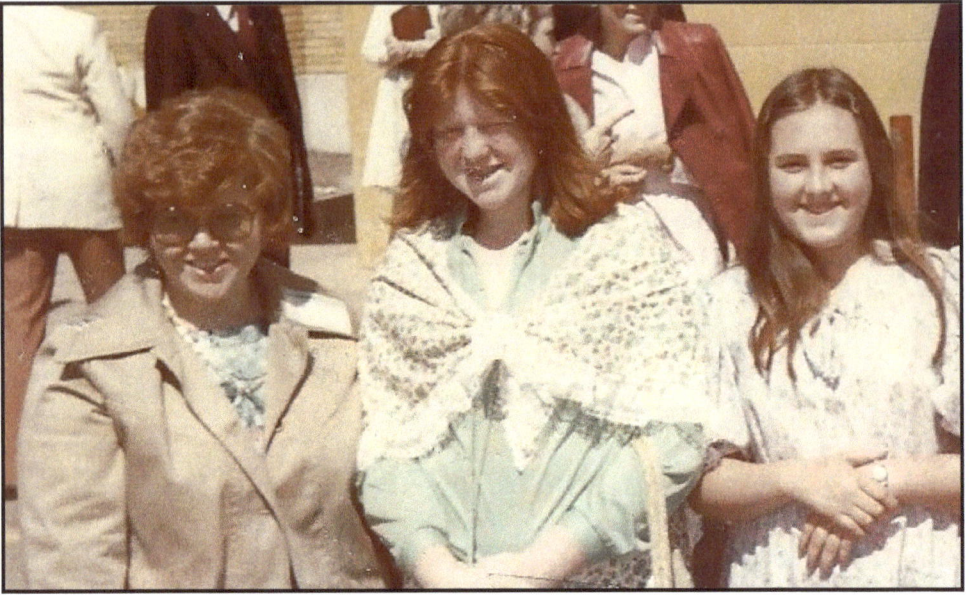

Gloria Clover, Danice Clover and Debbie Cole
at the Ark. City Junior High, 1977.

Mom would always make up songs while we were in the car or on the church bus.

She would sing,

"It's cold, so cold in Kansas.
You can freeze to death in Kansas.
But we don't care about the cold, cold air.
'Cause there's lots of love in Kansas."

She also wrote a song to the tune of Janis Joplin's "Oh, Lord Won't You Buy Me a Mercedes Benz. Mom's version was called "Oh, Lord won't you help me Make it Through the Day." I don't remember all of it but it went something like this:

Oh, Lord won't you help me make it through the day.
Guide me in the things I do and in the things I say.
My Spirit is so willing but my flesh is oh so weak.
Oh, Lord won't you give me a little of your strength.
Oh, Lord won't you help me let my light shine…

She really was a very creative person. She loved giving ideas to other people and letting them run with it, and she never worried about who got the credit.

After Mom retired from teaching, she decided to learn to play the piano. She said she had played the steel guitar when she was younger, but I never heard her play. I delighted in her piano playing and gave her a Roy Orbison song book in an attempt to try and repay her for all those lessons and songbooks she had purchased for me.

I write songs. I write poems. I'm writing this book. That's how I cope. I wrote Mom a song while she could still respond. I entitled it:

Don't Let Go Of Me.

Don't let go of me, Don't let go

If I should lose my grip, promise you won't let go of me

Riding my bike with the training wheels off

For the very first time

Afraid I'd fall and skin my knee

But Mom was running right beside me and

She heard my plea,

Please don't let go of me

Don't let go of me, Don't let go

If I should lose my grip, promise you won't let go of me

Her body failed and legs so weak

She could no longer stand

So scared she'd fall and break a knee

I held her up and took her hand to give her strength

And then I softly heard her plea

Don't let go of me, Don't let go

If I should lose my grip, promise you won't let go of me

      I got to share it with her one Sunday morning, while everyone else was at church. We cried together and held each other. I've sung it through one time since I shared it with her without crying. Oh, how I love that woman. I can't begin to describe in words what she means to me.

After she passed, I added this to the song;

I know you've promised you'd be here for me

But so did Mama now she's gone

As far as I can see

Don't let go of me, Don't let go

If I should lose my grip, Lord please don't let go of me

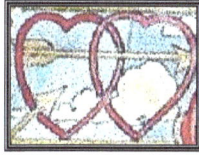

Chapter Eleven: Her Diagnosis

Mom started becoming concerned about the possibility of mercury in her system from a situation with a tooth. So she started documenting her visits to doctors and dentists.

On January 1, of 2005, Mom had a bagel for breakfast and chipped her tooth. This resulted in a visit to Mom's dentist in Wichita, Kansas. She returned to the dentist in February for preparation for a crown.

Mom wrote in her journal:

"on the 27th was this wonderful verse: This life that I live now, I live by faith in the Son of God, who loved me and gave his life for me. I refuse to reject the grace of God. Galatians 2:20.
On March 1, I got my crown on the tooth I broke January 1.
On the 31st, Terry Schivo (brain-damaged lady) died after 13 days of no food/water; it's been in the media a lot and very controversial.
On the 6th (April, 2005) I broke another tooth on an antacid tablet. I went to the dentist on the next day; I'll need another crown-$1200.
We came home on the 31st, our 1st day of being retired again. (May, 2005).
June, 2005. I had my ears washed out for the 1st time on the 1st; I couldn't hear and they felt strange.
September 2005: My gift to myself on my 65th birthday is go on a diet and rejoin T.O.P.S. (Taking Off Pounds Sensibly). Now I'm on Medicare, PTL (Praise The Lord).
Danice and I swam on the 22nd, the 1st day of fall, latest we've ever swam outside. I stayed home on the 26th. My chest and back were really hurting. Stayed home most of the day-not feeling good. Hurt the next day, too but not as bad. Went to the doctor on the 28th- esophogitis, and maybe ulcer.

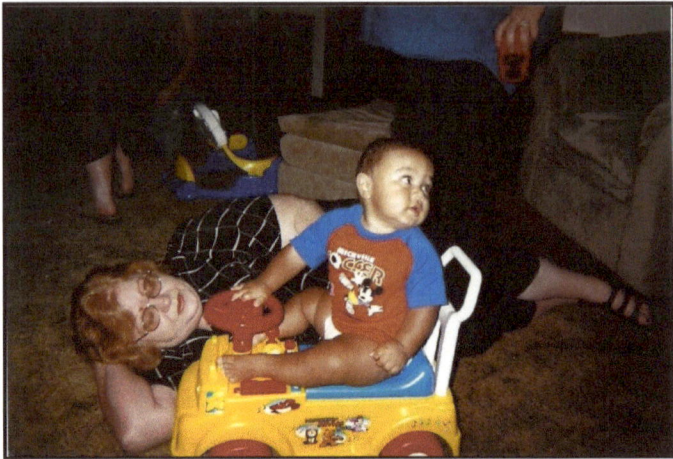
Mom & Gabe

Mom could always be found on the floor with the kids. She would get at their eye level and play. Gabe would want to ride her back like she was a pony, and before you could say, "Mom, that's going to hurt your back," she was on all fours, sounding like a horse.

> *October, 2005: Gabriel took 4 steps by himself. I began teaching in the after school program at Roosevelt on the 10th. I had a scope done at Winfield Hospital to look at my esophagus; it looked very good which makes me wonder about my heart because I had such pains in my chest and no energy at all last week.*
> *I went to the doctor on the 27th-had an EKG. Doctor said I had sugar diabetes and would have to go on medicine.*
> *"Thank you Lord for fellowship and beautiful weather."*

Amyotrophic lateral sclerosis is difficult to diagnose early because it may appear similar to several other neurological diseases. Tests to rule out other conditions may include:

- **Electromyogram.** This test measures the tiny electrical discharges produced in muscles. A fine wire electrode is inserted into the muscles that your doctor wants to study. An instrument records the electrical activity in your muscle as you rest and contract the muscle. This test is mildly uncomfortable for most people.
- **Nerve conduction study.** For this test, electrodes are attached to your skin above the nerve or muscle to be studied. A small shock is passed through the nerve to measure the strength and speed of nerve signals.

64

- **MRI.** Using radio waves and a powerful magnetic field, MRI can produce detailed images of your brain and spinal cord. It involves lying on a movable bed that slides into a tube-shaped machine, which makes loud thumping and banging noises during operation. Some people feel uncomfortable in the confined space.
- **Spinal tap (lumbar puncture).** This test analyzes the fluid surrounding your brain and spinal cord (cerebrospinal fluid). You typically lie on your side with your knees drawn up to your chest. A local anesthetic is injected in an area over your lower spine to reduce any discomfort from the procedure. Then a needle is inserted into your spinal canal, and fluid is collected.
- **Blood and urine tests.** Analyzing samples of your blood and urine in the laboratory may help your doctor eliminate other possible causes of your signs and symptoms.
- **Muscle biopsy.** If your doctor believes you may have a muscle disease rather than ALS, you may undergo a muscle biopsy. In this procedure, a small portion of muscle is removed while you're under local anesthesia and is sent to a lab for analysis. (Mayo 2008)

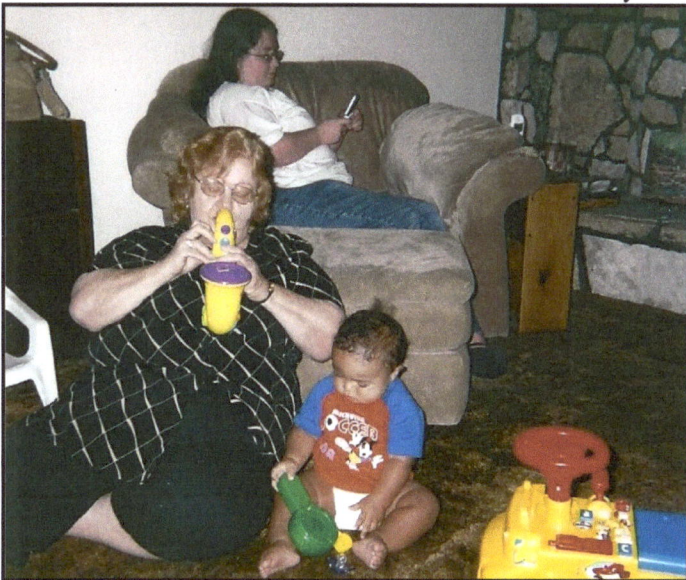

Mom, her granddaughter Christine and her great-grandson, Gabriel.

November, 2005, Holly's been accepted to Texas A & M grad school. I went to the dietician and diabetes educator on the 2nd and got a meter to monitor my diabetes. Sure hate to have to do this and learn that it will only get worse.

December, 2005. (My brother) Tom called- our cousin in KC died. Had heart problems, swollen feet and heart murmur. I have those last 2 things. I had a Dr. appt- he said I looked better physically, emotionally, etc, than he'd ever seen me. Made me feel good.
March 2006, I've lost 25 pounds so far. I was elected leader of TOPS on the 7th for next year. Got a chipped tooth filled. Danice and I played in a Scrabble Tournament; I won first place and she was 2nd.
April 2006. I had part of a crown come out of a front tooth. I went to the dentist on the 6th and got the crown put back on. We had supper at Danice's and an Easter Egg Hunt. All of our kids, grandkids and great- grandchild were there. Holly and Gabe were at Danice's on the 29th-I heard him say "Grandma" for the 1st time.

We started having concerns when her speech started slurring. The internet can be a wonderful thing, but it can also convince you that you have every disorder known to mankind. Mom, being the constant reader, began to narrow down her symptoms. It did not look good. No book, no website, nor doctor can tell you how to prepare for what ALS does. She started searching on line and started ordering books. One of the first was a book about ALS. (Mitsumoto, 2009) It seemed to describe the many symptoms and pains she was having.

Worldwide, ALS occurs in one to three people per 100,000. An inherited form of the disease occurs in 5 to 10 percent of the cases. But in the vast majority of cases, doctors don't yet know why ALS occurs in some people and not in others.

ALS often begins with muscle twitching and weakness in an arm or leg, or with slurring of speech. Eventually, ALS affects your ability to control the muscles needed to move, speak, eat and breathe. (Mayo)

Mom found a website called rob@everydayisprecious.com. As of this writing, Marcy Payne lost her struggle with ALS. Her husband Rob Payne is a writer and kept a daily post of ways to help people with ALS and their own struggle. Mom read it faithfully while she was able and was so appreciative of the scriptures and faith they show on the website. Rob Payne had also helped design a blinking system that he and his wife used to communicate. Dividing the alphabet into three rows of letters.

66

"March 2008: Goals for the month: Lose 5 lbs. by staying on 1200 calories a day and exercising at least 30 minutes a day. Get over this sinus/allergy problem. My teeth on the left side (opposite of where I had one pulled) started aching. ..the clinic called and told me that the CT scan said I had chronic sinusitis and prescribed an antibiotic which I am to take for 30 days. Maybe I'll finally get well. I couldn't sleep, felt dizzy, sick at stomach and anxious. I'm not taking any more of that medicine.*

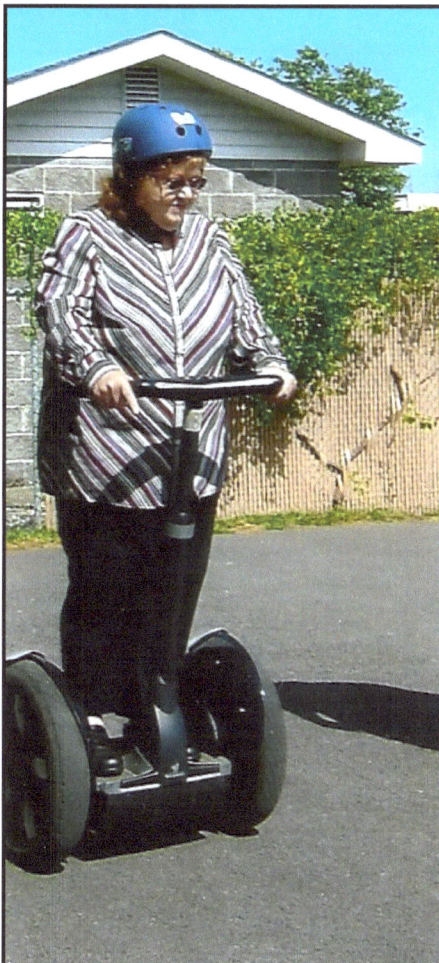

Mom was usually up for anything. Here she is riding a Segue at Branson in 2007. She also convinced me to join her on a helicopter ride in Branson when I was a teenager, and she made me sit on the seat closest to the edge with no door!

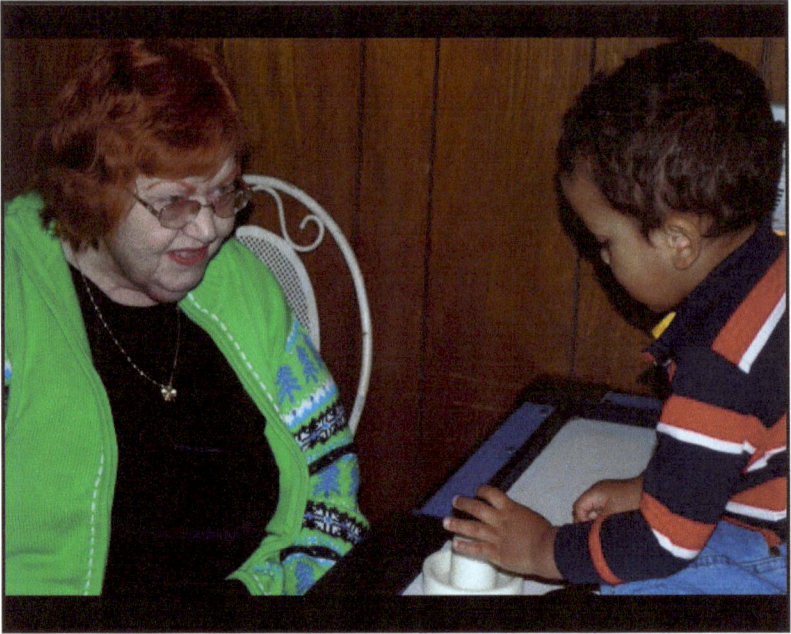

Mom and her great-grandson Noah playing Air Hockey.

We were always giggling at inappropriate times. She'd get tickled, and I'd get tickled, and we would have to leave the room -- we were laughing so hard. One time during a Sunday night church service, we got tickled. Sometimes it would be because Mom sang a little bit monotone. If she started a song in the car, which she did often, as we were growing up, she sounded fine. But in church, if some song got too low or high, she would stay on the previous note. She knew that this would make me giggle if it happened more than once in the same song.

That particular Sunday evening in the right hand side of the auditorium at church, we were singing a song, and she knew I had giggled. She started giggling, and we both tried to stop laughing. It got worse until we were both in tears. Finally she stood up and walked out to the foyer to gather her composure she came back in the back door on the left side of the auditorium, where we never ever sit. We could not even remain in the same pew without busting out.

After the service, some very concerned brothers and sisters in church asked if Dad was okay. They saw us both crying and knew something must have happened to him. We both answered that he was fine and were so embarrassed that our giggles to tears had caused others concern.

During the early part of discovering what ALS was and whether she had it, I noticed that her laughter was almost unstoppable. It wasn't the same kind of giggling we had done before. I knew something wasn't right.

She started getting rid of all household cleaners and any aerosol cans. This included anything like hairspray, deodorant, non-stick pan spray, furniture polish and even Windex. A few months later, she started tossing anything with MSG, Aspartame or any toxic ingredient.

"April 2008 Goals: Same as last month, stay on 1200 calories each day and lose 5 lbs. and get over this sinus/allergy problem. On Monday I went to the Dr. and ENT in Wichita. He said I had a polyp and blockage on both sides and needed to have sinus surgery. He ran a scope down my nose and could see my throat and said it looked okay. Another doctor would need to state that my health was okay for surgery, and he thought I might need a C-T scan of the brain to see if I had had a stroke, which could be causing the slurred speech. Danice got my prescription filled which should stop the drainage- almost $100. She said it was my Mother's Day gift. She had one of her classes pray for me. I'm hoping the medicine will clear up my throat and pray that I haven't had a stroke."

"May Goals: lose 5 lbs, have brain scan; sinus surgery? 2008: My left arm hurt all day which really concerns me. I was really feeling bad and get so emotional. I had an e-mail from a niece in California so I know the word is spreading that I don't feel well. I was breathless walking out to the store and left arm really hurting, so I'm wondering if it's my heart now... I have a sinus infection again. On Thursday I went to the doctor. I had a chest x-ray and an EKG in preparation for sinus surgery. Monday I am scheduled to have a brain scan (to see if I have had a stroke) and throat scan. On Saturday I had gotten choked on a baby aspirin and Jake had to give me the Heimlich maneuver, so they'll think I'm really in a bad way.

"On Monday the 20th, I had a brain scan and throat scan (C-T) at the hospital to see if I have had a stroke and if something is wrong with my throat. They used iodine, which concerned me, but I did okay."

69

"On the way to the zoo, the doctor's nurse called and said they'd gotten my c-t test results and I have not had a stroke and am okayed to have surgery. I called to try to cancel it but didn't get a response. The nurse from the ENT Dr. called and they have to get confirmation for surgery from the doctor which they don't have yet.

"I was swinging while holding Noah and fell out of the swing. It was funny but embarrassing.

June 2008: *I lost my record of the first 10 days but during this time I learned that my ENT Dr. is postponing my surgery until at least August and I'm no better. Sometimes I think there is something besides allergy/sinus wrong with me I am so tired of it.*

On the 21st, the first day of summer we went to the family reunion in Wagoner. There were about 35 there. It was fun. It was emotional for me not being able to talk very well and knowing everyone was wanting to hear how I sounded. Ever since I've had trouble talking, my emotions have been very difficult to control; I cry easily but also laugh uncontrollably. I sure hope that I can be well again.

I called another doctor at Holly's encouragement and he said if I have vocal cord paralysis it would never get better. That was discouraging. He set up an MRI of my brain and left shoulder for the next day. I couldn't lay on my back for the brain scan so just had the shoulder scan.

August 2008 Goals, Lose at least 5#.

Aug.1, Jake and I went to Ponca City Hospital where I had a spinal tap, which was very uncomfortable...had to lay flat on my back for 4 hours. On the 2nd, I had another spine MRI, I hope, but I'm worried about what they will say...... ..my voice seems to be getting worse, it scares me that I'll get to where I can't talk.

...the twitching is on my chin, around my mouth, and on my nose for the first time-plus on my arms and legs and back. Dr. called and said tests showed that my problems were not caused by my spine or diabetes ..so it is looking for sure like ALS. I've strongly suspected it all along but it still is frightening. Norma called and I just cried...Dear God please don't let it be ALS.

70

Hazel and Dorothy called today. I love my sisters and nieces and all of my family so much. Terry sent me a card with "Hope" on it. I'm having lots of contractions in my legs and around my mouth.

I fell out of my chair while Evelyn and I were playing Scrabble and couldn't get up because of my left arm. I had to call Jake.
We left for KU Medical Center. Aug. 11, I met with 2 doctors and 2 students and they did several tests; my left arm and hand were incredibly weak. They took my blood and ruled out Lyme disease. I had the electric current test and then the needle test on my left arm, hand and leg and then the diagnosis I had dreaded---

I Have ALS.

I cried most of the way home…I feel like I've had my death notice.
I will fight and do what I can. We ate at McDonald's at noon and Steve (the owner hugged me.)

Amyotrophic Lateral Sclerosis or ALS is often called Lou Gehrig's disease after Lou Gehrig, the famous New York Yankees baseball player who was diagnosed with ALS in the 1930s. ALS is a neurological disease that attacks the nerve cells responsible for controlling voluntary muscles. With ALS, eventually all muscles under voluntary control are affected…patients lose strength and ability to move their arms, legs and body.

When muscles in the chest fail, patients end up using a ventilator to breath and most people with ALS die from respiratory failure. It's a frustrating disease for both patients and doctors. There are no clear risk factors in about 90 to 95 percent of all cases…and no cure. Usually ALS patients die within 3 to 5 years from the onset of symptoms. However about 10 percent of patients survive 10 or more years. (ICYOU)

Early signs and symptoms of ALS include:
- Difficulty lifting the front part of your foot and toes (footdrop)
- Weakness in your leg, feet or ankles
- Hand weakness or clumsiness

- Slurring of speech or trouble swallowing
- Muscle cramps and twitching in your arms, shoulders and tongue

The disease frequently begins in your hands, feet or limbs, and then spreads to other parts of your body. As the disease advances, your muscles

become progressively weaker until they're paralyzed. It eventually affects chewing, swallowing, speaking and breathing. (ninds,2008)

"There's nothing good about ALS, but it has made me so much more aware of how awesome our Lord is and how he has blessed me with the most wonderful Family and friends anyone could have." Gloria Clover

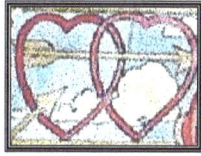

Chapter Twelve: Her Treatment

I called a number in Colorado about finding a dentist to pull my teeth with mercury...a man called back and told me about a place in Tex. It would cost about $10,000 but I feel it's my only hope. I decided to do it and liquidated my stock. It might be a total waste of money, it's probably a shot in the dark but I've got to try. I feel like it's my last and only chance to live.

The ALS nurse came by on Thursday. She was real nice. She suggested I get a feeding tube, large straw and bend my chin down when I swallow. She said not to have surgery unless absolutely necessary. I did not reach my goal of losing 5#

My speech has gotten much worse and it's getting harder to get out of chair; I have lots of facilitations all over and my left arm is almost useless.

September, 2008

Goal: Get mercury removed from my system and get a feeding tube put in.

Holly, Danice and boys came out. Evelyn came out and when I was going back into the house I fell again and Jake, Danice & Chet had to get me up. I guess I'm going to have to stop wearing sandals. Jake has been wonderful to me.

Now I'll be afraid to go anywhere by myself.

On September 6, 2008, we left for Marble Falls , Texas. I had read about mercury removal from several books and made a call to Colorado Springs, Colorado and learned only about two weeks ago of a clinic scheduled for the 8th. It took us about 12 hours to get there. After we checked in at the motel, we ate at a nearby café' and the cashier told us the dentist I was going to had saved her daughter's life. That was encouraging.

The next day a man at church once again told us that the Dr. was one of the best dentists in Texas. That evening all the people met at the dentist's office to "meet and greet." there were people from Oregon, Wyoming, Colorado, Wisconsin, Florida, Georgia, Hong Kong, Australia and of course, Kansas. The dentist office waiting room was decorated like the inside of a beautiful home with lovely sofas, tables, chairs, and pictures. I thought my niece Lezlie, who is skilled in decorating, would have approved.

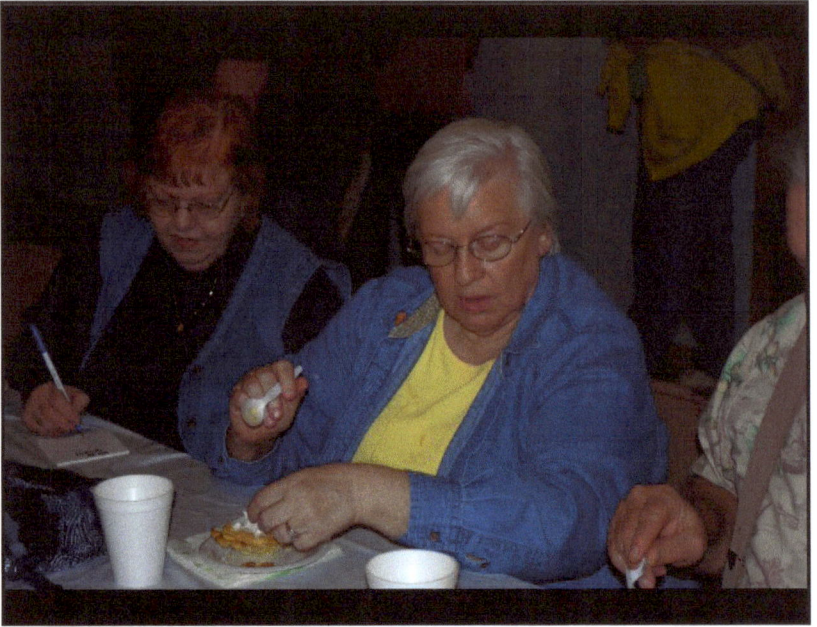

Gloria Clover and Virginia Vick.

Mom was unable to speak but could still write, consequently she always had a note pad or white board nearby to communicate.

October, 2008 Goals: go back to T.O.P.S, Lose 5 #, Feeding tube? I cooked beans and baked potatoes for Gibson's, Sweet's, Holly's family, Evelyn and us.

Jake sold his trailer yesterday and gave the money to help with Dale's truck payment. I went to McDonalds with Jake for breakfast for the first time since the 1st of July. Jake put handles by my bed, bath, and backdoor. Yeah. Dayna was up to help with Gabe; we played a game of Scrabble. Danice took an abandoned kitten home from the barn. They named it Gracie.

On the 6th, I went to Dr. about my arm. A friend of Danice's in Texas wrote letters to many of the KS Politicians about Medicare helping more with ALS.

Chet was 51 on the 7th; Danice had us, Evelyn, Holly and boys out for supper. I went to Tops and weighed in and started crying and couldn't talk and doing the wailing I do. So I left. I thought I was

74

over the crying. We had really nice letters from Dale. Hazel called and I cried; I'm so disappointed I'm crying again. Two technicians from Wichita came down to check out the sleeping machine; one of them prayed for me. She said her brother died with ALS; it was discouraging and I cried. Evelyn and Danice came to play Scrabble. I can barely talk at all and can tell I'm getting weaker; it's very discouraging.

Church gave us a check for $2500 from the benefit. We took food by Bonnie Martin's. We got flu shots and found out they had 20 units of Mercury. I feel like ALS is really attacking my face and bladder. I had a dream where I said I had ALS. Acceptance? Noah was 2 today. We stopped at ALS office in Wichita and got a bed rail, walker, portable stool, and bath seat.

Chelation Therapy is a technique of taking mercury from the body, primarily the teeth. Some dentists in the Midwest still put mercury in fillings. When you Google the phrase "chelation therapy" you get over 470,000 results as of this writing. It promises everything from blocking the absorption of Calcium, to improving Cell Energy Production, to reducing Free Radical Activity in the blood. (holisticonline.com)

But the American Heart Association and other medical and scientific groups have spoken out against this treatment. (American heart.org). After much review, they have concluded that the Benefits claimed for this form of therapy are not scientifically proven. (American, 2010).

Chelation therapy is administering a man-made amino acid called EDTA into the veins. EDTA is an abbreviation for ethylenediamine tetra acetic acid. It's marketed under several names including, Edetate, Disodium, Endrate and Sodium Versenate. EDTA is most often used in cases of heavy metal poisoning (lead or mercury). That's because it can bind these metals, creating a compound that can be excreted in the urine.

When the medical world offers you no hope whatsoever, you look elsewhere. We started going to Whole Foods stores and getting organic everything. Organic lean meat, organic frozen meals, hummus, anything with protein. We even switched to an organic, non-toxic hair color.

One of Mom's favorite resources was a book called, *Eric is Winning*. The author, Neal Rouzier, MD. He states that Eric has survived ALS for over 14 years. Having first been diagnosed in 1993, he was able to gather a great deal of information about ALS and developed a program of how to beat it. (Rouzier, 2010)

The book emphasizes eliminating toxins from your body from three main sources: dental fillings containing mercury, accumulated toxic heavy metals and any pathogens in your colon and/or bloodstream such as fungi or Lyme disease. (Eric, 2010)

October 29th, we went to Tulsa to pick out a communication device at T.U. It's a hard decision. I'm starting to have difficulty getting up from stool and chairs. I've had cramps in my right leg (around ankle) for the last two nights; it worries me that I'll get unable to walk.
November, 2008 Goal: Vitamin C drip and Feeding tube?
I had terrible leg cramps and its scares me that I could be losing the use of my legs. Holly brought me some organic drinks, meat and an air purifier. We spent the day at the Garvey Center in Wichita; talked with several people and gave blood and urine and hair sample and received Vitamin C drip and acupuncture on my ear. Danice gave me her Mac laptop to type on and it speaks out the words. I had to wear a deal on my finger all night to measure my oxygen.

She began taking large amounts of vitamin C. Then the intravenous Vitamin C drips began while she was in Texas, receiving the Chelation Therapy. She continued receiving Vitamin C intravenously until she could no longer travel to get them. She also tried to get out in the sun at least thirty minutes a day to increase the body's absorption of vitamin D. She researched that sunshine is a natural anti-depressant, and when she couldn't get outside to get vitamin D, she took vitamin D.

On the fourteenth I had a stress test on the treadmill. Holly helped me dress and undress. I did much better than I thought so I should soon be getting scripts for Rilutek and Lithium which has stopped the progress of ALS in mic. Hope it will work for me

Our acapella group, Revival, came up to Arkansas City for a Jeans & Beans Benefit concert. Mom and Dad have traveled to hear me sing since I was in High School. From our ladies church group, Joyful Sounds, to our quartet in college, New Creation, to our time with Acappella, no family could have been as supportive of our music, as my family has been.

76

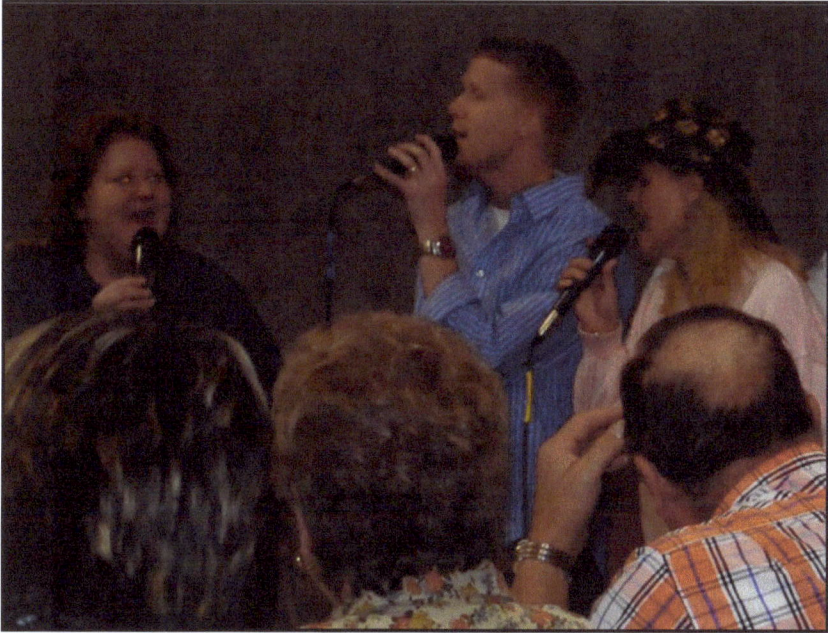

Danice, Craig Hayes and Donja Hayes Cary
at the Jeans and Beans Benefit Concert for Mom.

November 17th - I can barely type with my left hand; the little finger sticks out; the index and middle finder seem to be swollen and are bent. On the 21st, we went to MDA doctor at 9:00 and the Garvey doctor at 2:30 and then had pinochle at the Vick's. It was a long day but MDA is going to give us $2000 to help with the communication device. On the 24th we ate at Pizza Hut; I saw Kay; she hugged me and I cried. A chair easy-lift came.

We had Thanksgiving at our house; we ate at noon. Dayna, Jerry, Tom, Glenda, Chrissy, Evelyn, Danice & Chet, Holly and the boys, Kay and Dallas and Jake and I were there. I kept thinking it might be the last time I can have it. We had a wonderful meal, played games and visited.

On Friday the Cole's came by. Danice, Chet and Holly and the boys came by. Danice and Chet came by on the 29th and helped put up the tree and decorations.

January 2009: Goal: Feeding Tube; Lose 3#-DID BOTH

On the first, we ate at the steak house for our 47th Anniversary. Danice and Laura came by and played a game of Scrabble. On the 5th, I smoked up the house with a pan of meat; I thought the burner was on off and it was on high. I had a rough night last night; my nose was plugged up and throat felt full so I didn't sleep well. On the 9th the lady from the communication device came again and Clara came by and visited. The Cole's had us and the Vick's over for supper and cards. This was about my 3rd night to have throat/coughing problems causing little sleep.

On the 11th, The repertory therapist came by and traded my mask for a full mask. Danice came by with lunch and refried beans. We bought burial spots at Parker Cemetery. I had blood taken at the hospital for KU; it's about all I can do to walk to the lab. It got much colder on the 23rd and sleeted some so I didn't go anywhere. After couples' pinochle here, I was coming to the house and I fell hard on the concrete and they called Chet to get me up. My head bled and I have a knot on my head.

After church and lunch Sunday we headed to KU med center in Kansas City. They provided us with a motel room. About 2 a.m. I got up to go to the bathroom and fell between the stool and tub. It really hurt. Jake had to get the manager to help me get up. We saw a team of people and they want me to get a neck brace and use a walker all the time and for Jake to get training on how to get me up. On the 29th we set the date for my feeding tube. It will be Monday. On the 30th, the Vick's came by and picked us up and we went to Hewins; Norma fixed lunch-chicken and noodles; then we played cards.

On the last day of January, Danice came by and gave me a manicure, pedicure and shaved my legs. She also brought supper...We went to Olen's Medical for a neck brace...We went to the Garvey Center and saw the doctor. They stuck me 3 times and couldn't get a vein so we came home. Jake felt really bad on the 28th-mumbling, not walking well. Danice, Dayna, Jerry, Holly, Dale and Chrissy were all here concerned about him.

Febuary,2009 Goals: Feeding tube, lose 3#, neck brace.

On the 2nd I went into the hospital and got a feeding tube. It hurt a lot more than I thought it would. We slept in recliners 3 nights.

Home Health Care came on the 4th and cleaned the dressing and taught us how to feed through it. My voice was much weaker today. I got choked on 2 pills real bad.

March 2009 Goals: write obit and letters to groups

Jake went to the doctor and found out he may have had a mild stroke (the kids were right). Tom and Glenda came, Stewarts came by. On the 7th, Daddy's birthday, Jake's mom died about 8:00 p.m. When Major left he took my hand and said, "I love you." On the 8th Jake *and Frieda made funeral arrangements for Elva and cleared out her room. We got her toilet riser, tv and lift chair. I didn't go to church; my feet and hand are swollen. Jaime Testerman brought flowers and Dean and Phyllis came by. Denise Wallace brought by 3 dishes. Later in the evening I fell in the living room and Jake and Dale had a hard time getting me up. Elva's memorial service was on Sat. at 11, There were lots of Venn's and Clover's. Tom and Glenda, Gerry and Bruce, and Mike and Tammy came. I went in a wheel chair for the first time. Danice sang.*

Don and Norma had us and Beth and Jeep over for cards. Don built a ramp to make it easier for me to get in and they had moved a big table into the living room and had a tall chair and cushion for me.

I rode the scooter out to the store and when I was coming back to the house it threw me down to the ground. Danice got back from Tulsa and came by. I didn't make it to church and couldn't stop crying. Danice came and stayed with me and ate with us and gave me a manicure and pedicure. Our electric went out about 7:30. Days are long without electric or cable. They finally got the electric back on at 7:30 at night. Cole's had us over and she made guac and refried beans for me and brought a chair I'd liked from the farm.

April 2009, Goals: Finish letters; lose 5#, start new treatment

On the 1ˢᵗ, we finally got cable back on. It's getting to where I can hardly eat. I can barely walk; my calves feel stiff. Laura and Jaime came by. Dayna came by and I was asleep; she called later and was crying because she missed me. Kate Darby came by and cleaned. On the 11ᵗʰ we went to the DeVault's in Broken Arrow. 26 were there. I did pretty good until we started to leave and then I cried and cried. Bick kissed me on the head several times and said he loved me.

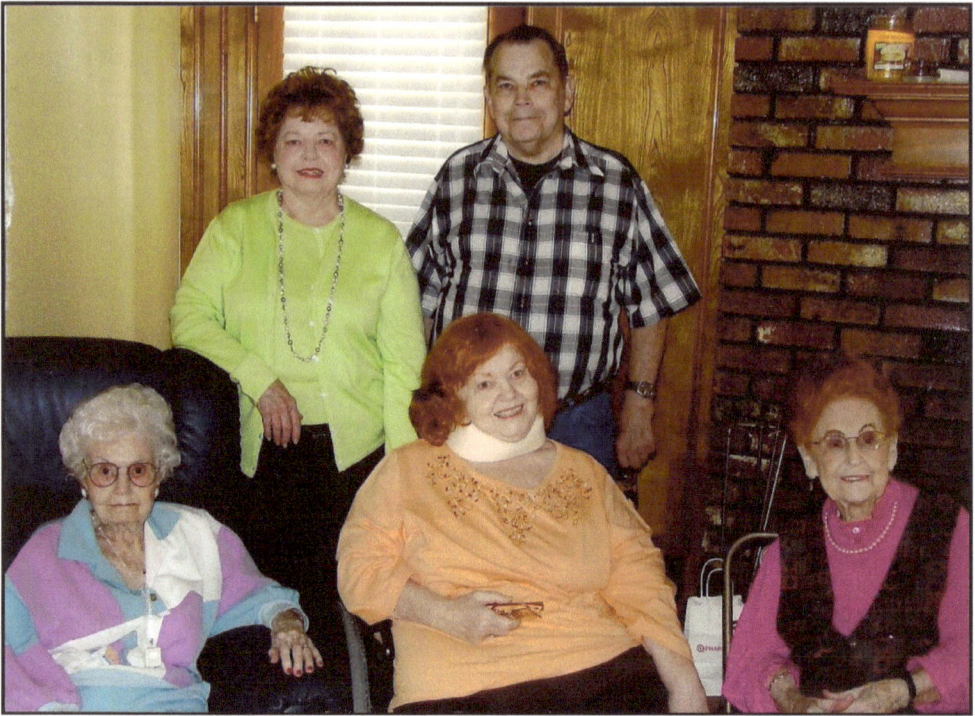

April 11, Tammy & Mike DeVault's home in Broken Arrow, Oklahoma.
Hazel, Gerry, Mom, Tom and Dorothy

April 20, we left at 4 a.m. for KU med center. My air was down to 27 and they advised calling hospice-very upsetting. We were both exhausted by the time we got home. Hospital bed now. I began having sponge baths instead of getting into the tub for a shower. It was scaring me. Vern came out to talk about Hospice; Danice and Chet were here. On the 23rd the Cole's came out; she brought pudding and custard. Sharon cut my hair.....Jake and I both fell as we were getting ready for bed; I hit the couch. On the 29th Holly and Noah came by; she found me on the floor. I fell on my face.

When Holly found Mom face down on the floor, she yelled,

"Grammy are you all right?"

She got her up and Mom asked for paper and a pen. "Of course I'm all right, I was getting a closer look at the carpet," she wrote sarcastically.

Friends and family members kept asking why Hospice or Home Health had not been brought in to assist Dad. Mom was a very modest person and did not want anyone to have to care for her. At our insistence they finally started receiving help. A wonderful Hospice nurse named Chrissy started coming.

At first, Mom would only allow her to take her vital signs and straighten the house. This sweet nurse was humble and helpful and eventually won Mom's heart. She was so gentle and so kind that I am still grateful today for all she did.

Mom always said a redhead should never go gray. "Gray and red don't go together," she'd complain. So she wrote me a note and asked, "Do I need color?" I had to respond honestly, "Yes, the gray is peeking through." I knew what this would mean. As difficult as it was for Dad and I to shampoo her hair, Chrissy and I would have to find a way to color her hair while she was in her wheelchair, without soaking her. Chrissy brought a portable hair tub from Hospice and we filled it with air like a little child's swimming pool and it surrounded her neck and had a tube that went to a bucket on the floor. Dad did understand how important a woman's hair color is, was, and always will be. We finally finished the process, using a natural hair color we found at a Health Food store and mom was thrilled with the result. It was important to her, and therefore, important to me.

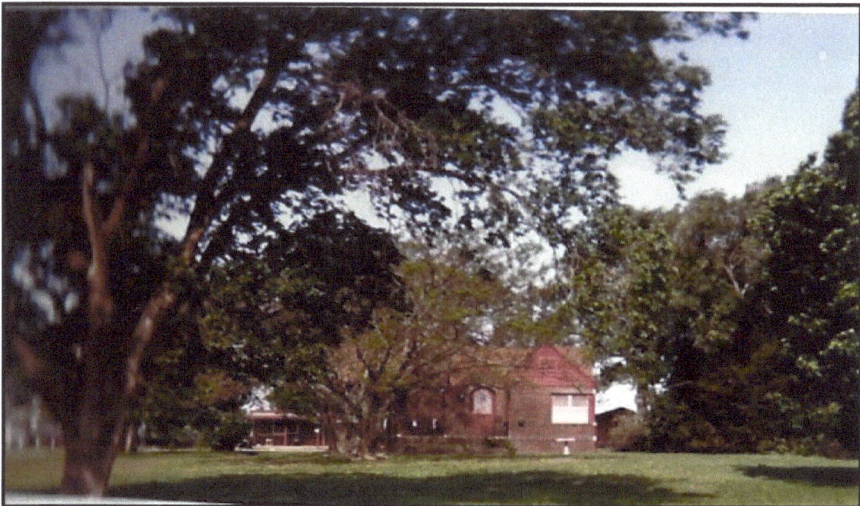

1996 Moving to 3225 N. Summit

81

I wanted to include one of Mom's actual journals. She began re-typing them and kept that up until July 2009 when she asked me to put on the computer the notes she had made. Here is her copy of May, 2009.

MAY, 2009

GOALS: LOSE 5#

We had rain and hail on the 1st. The Rt lady came. Danice came by. Holly and boys came out; they leave early in the morning for D.C. Evelyn came out. On the 2nd, Dayna and Jerry came up and Danice and Laura stopped by. We went to church on the 3rd and the Cole's had us and the Vick's over for cards. On the 5th, Jim Whitley finished working on the ramp. Julie, Danice, and Evelyn came by. Phyliss brought a vase of peonies. Holly called. Dale went to Dallas with his friend Phil. On the 5th, Jake ate with Herb It rained. Tresia and Danna brought supper. Danice came by. Her biopsy came back malignant. Evelyn came out. On the 6th, Chrissy was 27. Danice spoke at South haven. Evelyn didn't feel good. Jim Whitley and Dale Harms picked up limbs in the yard. Evelyn came out on the 7th; Danice came out and stayed quite awhile. Danice and Evelyn came by. Holly and boys are back. They came out on the 9th—glad to be back. Danice came by. Evelyn came out.On the 10th we had lunch here after church. We celebrated Chrissy's birthday and Mother's Dsy. My girls got me a framed picture of an embroidery of our last name We were all there, including Evelyn and Vern came by. Dayna gave me pens and.notepads and Chet gave me a dozen roses. Jake gave me a lawn chair. On the 11th Julie came. L:adies' pinochle was here. Danice received her 20 year pin.Dayna and Jerry came up. Virginia Hensley came by on the 12th. Danna and Tresia brought supper. Evelyn came out. On the 13th, holly, Danice and boys came out. Norma came by with custard. On the 14th, Virginia Hensley came by with pictures of Mason'. Danice came by twice. Jennies came by and played her violin. Kate and Evelyn were out. Jerry found out he had blockage; we sent money to them with Danice. On the 15th, Danice came by and then she and Chet came by. [   ]
On n the 16th, holly and boys came out; Danice and Evelyn came out. I didn't go to church on the 17th; Danice, Dale, holly and boys stayed with me. Dayna, Jerry, and Evelyn came by. Since the 15th, I haven't eaten. On the 18th, Julie, Danice and Evelyn came by. On the 19th, Virginia Hensley, Danice, and Evelyn came by. Jerry had 4 bypasses on the 21st. Jake ate with Herb and I had to go to the restroom and could not get up so I sat there for about an hour.
On the 20th, Clara came and brought a pie, Danice, Holly and boys and Evelyn came by. On the 21st Jake bought a handicapped van for $1000. Kate, Laura, Danice and Evelyn came by. On the 22nd Carolyn Johnson called. Danice, Laura, and Evelyn came by. On the 23rd, AEverone was here; ;I had an uti and they tried to get me in the van but that didn"t work.On the 24th, Gerry and Tammy came up and we all ate here. I didn't feel good at all. Julie, Danice and Holly were by on the 25th.Don and Norma came by. On the 26th, Tom and Glenda drove Dayna and Jerry home and then came up here. Dale began his new job at Caldemar. Evelyn was out twice and Danice 4 times. On the 27th. Virginia came by and danice and a nurse from hospice. On the 28th, danice, ginger. Evelyn. Holly and boys were out. On the 29th, danice and evelyn were out danice got me

---

82

The June journal entry was much shorter due to drastic changes in my mother's condition.

June 2009: I had a really nice letter from Dayna. Jake and Danice visited Dayna and Jerry he's in ICU. Evelyn and Julie stayed with me. Jerry was taken by ambulance to OKC with bleeding around his heart. Chet came by and gave me a gait belt.

On the 3rd, Danice went to OC to be with Dayna. Jerry had surgery and they said he probably won't make it. Tony Tipton died.

On the 5th Danice had pinochle here. I can't put the cards in the rack anymore. Chet sat with me during church time.

On the 17th Danice had surgery they think they got it all..Mary read to me..Danice, Laura and a lady from hospice came by, Kate and Evelyn. Rose Rice died. On the 19th, Jeri was 91.

This is the first time you can see mom's typing really start to deteriorate.

Evleyn was out; we had 3 hospice [eople, als nurse and two rt people. Ja ke went to Wichita to g e t a scooter and hoi s t; danice s a t with me. Dayna, mary, and ev el yn wer out 03on the 25th,d anic e, hilly and boy s,kate, vern bb2 n/urses asdnd 2 housecleansers were ougtu.

D anic ne got a no cvasncerr report from tyhte dr.

Mom asked me to try and type up her notes for her journal in July. The vital points were:

July 2009, on the 2nd, our Hospice nurse and housekeeper were by. Danice came by and helped wash my hair. Evelyn came out and Jerry is back in the hospital with pneumonia. Nurse brought me patches for drooling. On the 4th, Jill came, Loretta and Evelyn came by. Tom, Glenda and Kay came by . July 8, Jake and Dayna followed the ambulance to OKC, Jerry has a blood clot…

I tried to get out but the wheelchair was too high for the handicapped van. Dee & Frank Pinegar came from Texas to see me. Sandy Allen came by, Danice stayed with me while Jake went to be with Dayna while her husband Jerry had surgery to remove the rest of sternum and get rid of infection in wound. I fell while Danice & Holly tried to get me in my chair. Chet and Dale came to help and Tricia, Hospice nurse gave me morphine for should pain. Holly, Phil and boys came, Jill Winegar came with Dale.

July 16, It's getting harder for me to get in and out of my chair.

July 17, I fell again. Jake and Dale got me up and Vern and Ginger and a nurse came by.

83

July 28, Beth brought a casserole, cookies and tomatoes. Danice came out with Laura and got Holly a birthday gift and a baby gift for the Bossie's new boy.

August, 2009 Ron and Craig Hayes came by to visit. Chet sat with me during church.

We had a Scrabble party in the store for Danice's 45th Birthday. Denise Wallace, Julie Kratt, Mary Whitley, Jennifer and Kate Darby, Evelyn, Loretta Harms, and Sharon Ternes came. Everyone had a great time. We ordered pizza.

8-7 slept most of the day. Evelyn and Jill were out. Danice started back to school.

8-11 One year ago today I was diagnosed with ALS. I had 4 falls over the past week. We are starting to use the sling to move me from bed to chair and to wheelchair. Danice brought the boys by and Dale & Jill were here. They moved one of the teal couches to the store...the boys helped. Danice and Donja came over and played Scrabble.

8-24 Norma sat with me for 3 hrs. while Jake went to Wichita. Danice 1st night teaching at CCCC. 8-25 I can't reach farther than my botton lip and all my fingers are bent.

8-27 Rough day, Jake's right hand was paralyzed and he couldn't move me from the bed to chair. He's exhausted. Danice came and together they got me in the chair.

8-28 Jerry back to OKC to hospital. Evelyn came out to stay with me so Jake could go. Bob Ternes went with him to get Dayna's car there. Holly, Danice and the boys came out.

8-30 Chet sat with me during church and all ate here. Christine and Laura stopped by.

This is where Mom's journals end. She could no longer write or share what she wanted to say about each day.

One day, I remember her asking what it was like outside. She said it had been two weeks since she had seen the sunshine, so we got her in her wheelchair and outside in the sun with sunglasses on and a quilt. She couldn't believe the leaves were already changing. It was then, I realized things would not ever be the same. A season had passed, and she had not been able to leave her home. The house they lived in on Summit Street was not made for wheelchair access.

A dear friend, Jim Whitley, had created handicap ramps into the house and into the store; that's what we called the building behind the house, that had once been a western wear store. But the house had tight corners and Mom often tore the trim while trying to maneuver through the kitchen especially.

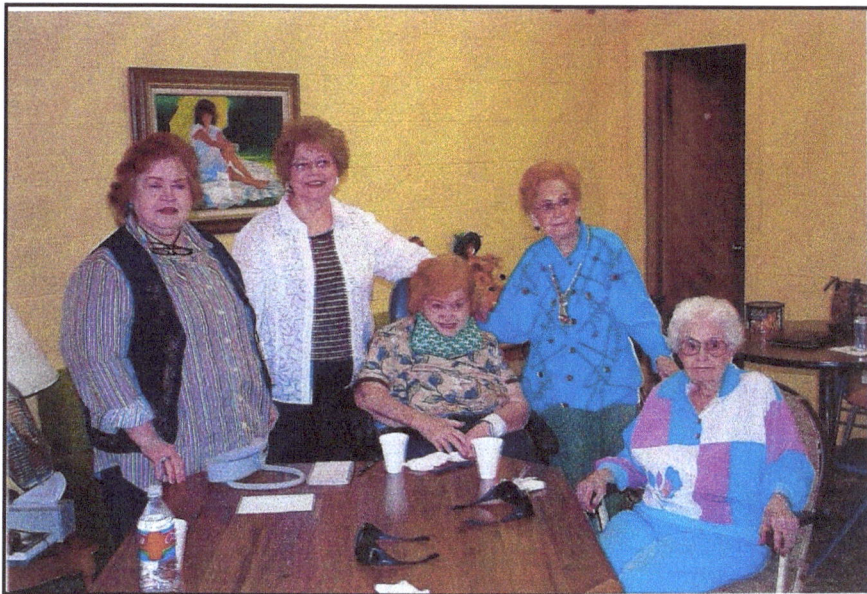

Aunt Evelyn, Aunt Gerry, Mom trying to smile,
Aunt Dorothy and Aunt Hazel.

The four walls of the living room were closing in around her and that's no way to live. I cried every time I left my parents' home. Praying for a miracle, I could not do as Mom had asked. She began asking for us to pray she would go home to Heaven. The morphine no longer had much effect on her pain. I prayed and begged and promised the Lord all I had if He would just restore her health.

Her hand became increasingly stiff. We tried splints on her fingers at her request. She thought if she could keep them from closing that they might keep working.

Gloria Clover was determined to find a cure for ALS. She kept track of current research as long as she was able. In her notes I found headings like:

"Studies confirm region of chromosome 9 linked to risk for amyotrophic lateral sclerosis August 30."
"Genetic variations on chromosome 9 have been identified that might have a role in the development of amyotrophic lateral sclerosis (ALS) and frontotemporal dementia."
"Findings in two separate Articles published Online First in The Lancet Neurology add to the evidence that a region of chromosome 9 is linked to a higher risk of ALS across multiple populations."

She wanted the entire family to read about ALS and to know what was coming.

"About 5-10% of ALS (also known as motor neuron disease or Lou Gehrig's disease) is hereditary. A few genes have been linked to ALS, but these explain only a small proportion of familial cases. The cause of the more common sporadic ALS remains largely unknown. Several recent genome-wide association studies (GWAS) have identified a number of possible susceptibility genes, but replication of these associations has not been successful in independent studies. In 2006, linkage between familial ALS and chromosome 9 was first identified in Scandinavian families. However, subsequent research has not revealed a disease-causing gene variant."

In the first Article, Bryan Traynor from the National Institutes of Health, USA, and international colleagues did a study to identify genetic risk factors for ALS in the Finnish population. The researchers found two genetic variations that contribute to risk of ALS. One was identified in the SOD1 gene, which has previously been associated with risk of ALS. The authors conclude: "The chromosome 9p21 locus is a major cause of familial ALS in the Finnish population." (physorg.com)

The number and chromosomes sounded like gobbledygook to me at first. But then when I realized approximately 10% of ALS is inherited, I started thinking about the symptoms. My sister, Dayna and I began wondering if we might inherit the disease and every cough and runny nose caused us to reflect on how Mom's symptoms started.

We still call each other when there is a special on television about ALS. We know more about it than we ever thought we would, and that still isn't much.

One of Mom's last trips to the Medical Center in Kansas City, the specialist told her to prepare for the last stage. They told her to get her house in order and make plans for her funeral.

Dad says she cried all the way home. They told them she might have six months left, and she would lose the ability to breathe and that resuscitation would be impossible. When the muscles can no longer push the air in and out of the lungs, breathing is a feat of Olympic strength.

Watching her fight for breath was heart wrenching. She stopped moving. She could no longer turn her head. She could not move a finger to write or point.

She asked us to pray she could go home to Heaven. I begged her not to ask us that. But then I realized, the cure for ALS would not come in her lifetime.

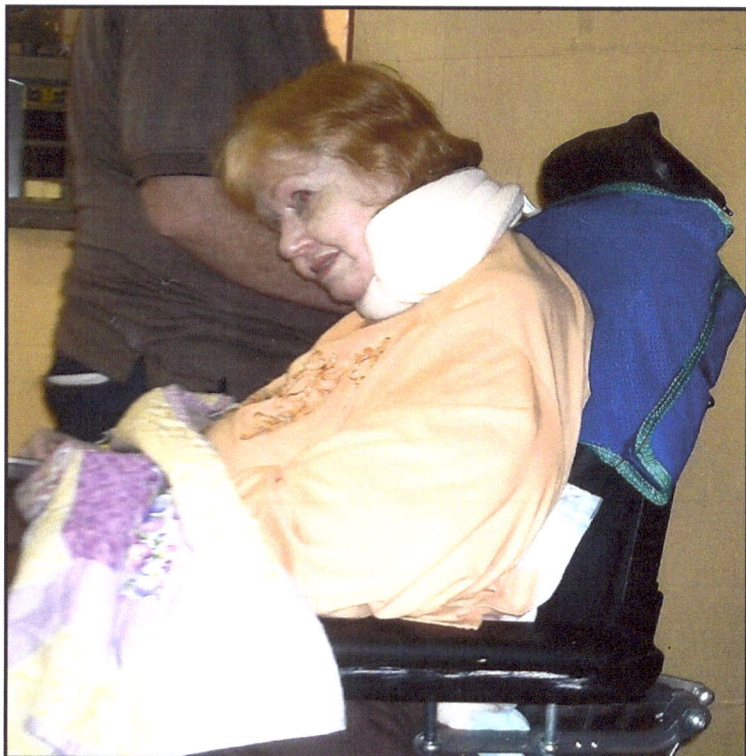

Dad called on Saturday morning, and said, "Your momma wants to see you." I ran out to their house, crying and scared, and when I saw her that day, her eyes said it all. They looked longingly at me, without being able to say a word. I knew she was ready to go.

I stayed and put lotion on her dry, swollen, still feet. Her toes were cold and though she never wore socks, I insisted on putting them on her feet. I cleaned her fingernails and held her hand. I walked into the kitchen several times to weep and wipe the tears and came back to her side.

My sister was in Oklahoma City with her husband who was in the hospital. I called her and told her it was time for her to come. She called her husband's brother to come to sit with him at the hospital.

I called my cousin Tammy from Tulsa and asked her to come on Sunday. I leaned on her so much during the last few months. She had lost her Mom, Wava, Mom's sister and also her father, Tinker, when she was a young adult, and she would listen when I could only cry.

I didn't sleep that night. I just kept praying.

Father, if it be your will, heal my momma. I know you can do all things, but I know my momma is ready to come home. I've been so blessed, Lord, but I don't think I can go through this. Lord, if you need her in Heaven today, then take her home to be with you. End her pain, bring her peace and help us all get through this. I love you, Lord. I know she is tired of hurting.

Your will be done, God. You knew loss after giving up Jesus for us. I can't comprehend sending your son for a sinner like me. But right now, my best friend, my momma can't speak, can't eat, and can't move. She doesn't want to live this way. So I beg you, heal her. You say it, and it will be so. I know you have the power and can do it. We will praise your name forever, regardless of what happens. You know what we want. We want her to be healed and to jump out of that hospital bed and light up the room and our corner of the world. But, you may have a hole in Heaven and need an organizer, a giver, a pinochle player, and the best momma you ever created. So, Father God, I give her to you. For you gave her to me, and I thank you.

Send your Holy Spirit to give us comfort and to relieve my momma of her pain. In your son, Jesus, I pray. Amen.

Dad called Sunday morning. He was fairly certain she wouldn't make it through the day. Her breathing became so shallow, and she could not close or open her eyes. They just stared out like she was looking at a new home. Within hours, she was with Jesus.

God gave her peace, and we knew she was ready. Her prayer is that we will all be ready to meet her as well.

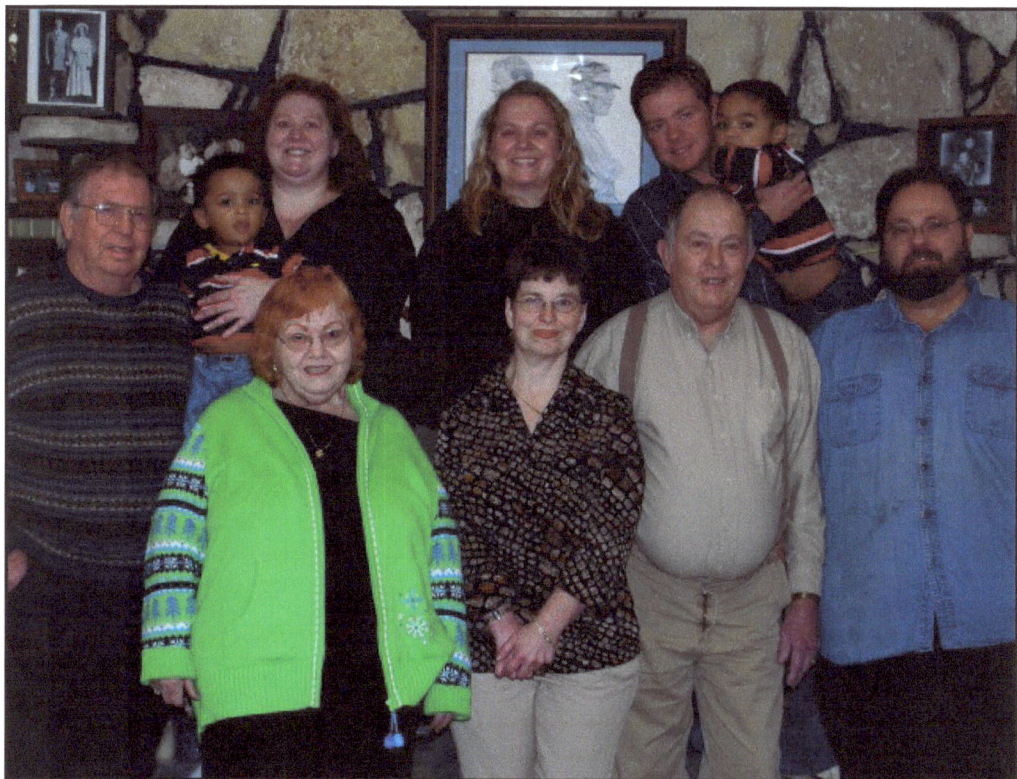

Back row: Jake Clover, Noah Harper, Danice Sweet, Holly Harper, Dale Beaty, Gabriel Harper
Front row: Gloria Clover, Dayna Gibson, Jerry Gibson and Chet Sweet. (Christmas 2008)

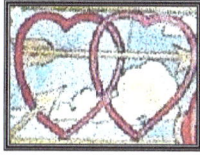

Chapter Thirteen: Her Legacy

Gloria Clover was an organizer. She could and did organize banquets for Senior Citizens on Thanksgiving, concerts for the Senior High School Students at church, card parties and gourmet pinochle clubs, and she also kept her house organized.

She kept her medicine cabinet in alphabetical order. Aspirin, Back aches, Colds… all the way to Zyrtec. No, I think that might have been in the A-allergy drawer, nevertheless, she was organized.

She would clean and reorganize the second shelf of every drawer on the second week of the month. On the third week of the month, she would sort and organize the third drawer of every cabinet, etc. It gave her pleasure to be organized.

After she retired, Mom came to my art room at one of the schools where I teach, and asked if she could organize it. I never turn down help, especially from my mother, so she came every Tuesday for one semester and started labeling and placing art supplies in tubs. The only problem was, she didn't know about all the art supplies. Rollers that apply ink to paper and wood are called brayers. I would have placed it under R for rollers or B for brayers. Mom placed it under I for ink, although they can also be used for paint. I still find boxes and tubs she labeled and I just grin. Rubber Leaf stamps are in the box marked Fall Decorations, not under stamps or leaves or ink or paint. We use leaf designs in times other than fall, but that is where she thought they belonged. She tackled any job, any drawer, any cabinet and could make sense out of it. When we moved to the country, I told her how overwhelmed I felt about moving after living in the same place for seventeen years. She said, "Tackle one box a day, and before you know it, you'll be done."

That's how she tackled ALS:

1. Research everything there is to know.

2. Do everything you can physically and mentally do to prepare and then pray.
3. Pray for your body, your mind, and your family and friends.
4. Pray for wisdom to create a system for expressing yourself when you can no longer speak.
5. Pray for a miracle.
6. Get your house in order.

So that's what we did. She created a blinking system. One blink for "yes," two for "no." She also instructed me to create charts that became like a flash card system. She wrote it out on notebook paper, and I created it on the computer. There was one for her different collars that supported her neck, one for communicating, and one for the blankets she preferred.

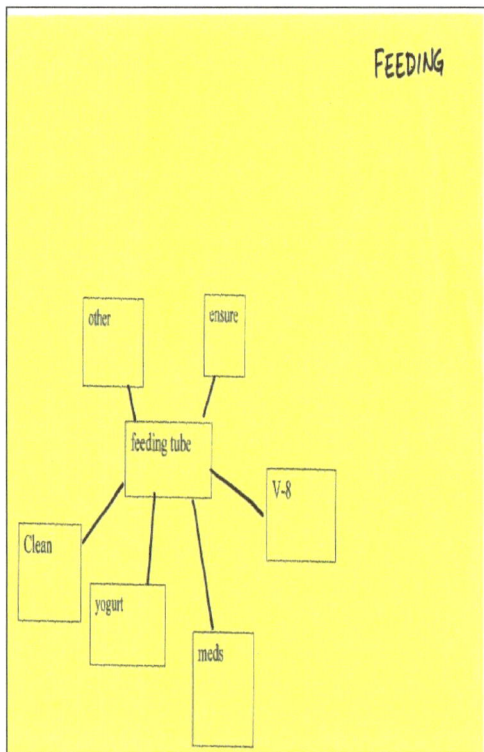

We revised it several times and practiced using it, knowing the time would come when she could not tell us what she needed. She would stare at the square she wanted, and I would point to it, and then she would nod or blink if it was correct. That was her greatest fear: *"Not being able to communicate and putting a burden on others to care for me."*

"Not death, but the process of dying," she said.

When Mom had to have a feeding tube put in, it was a whole new learning curve for all of us. She would often throw up, and be unable to swallow or cough. It became terrifying every time she began to choke. The doctors insisted that no one perform the Heimlich Maneuver because it could cause more damage. She had to learn to somehow work the liquid in her throat up out of her mouth with limited muscle control. We lost count of how many times Mom choked. As scary as it was for us, it must have been terrifying for her.

March 2009 Goals: write obit and letters to groups.
April, 2009 Goals: Finish letters: lose 5#; start treatment.

Over ninety red headed dolls decorated every nook and cranny of her home. Once you start collecting something, it multiplies like rabbits. Soon, anyone who saw a redheaded doll began giving them to Mom. She tried to pass that love of dolls to me, but it never took. Everyone who came to the service was asked to take a redheaded doll to remember Mom by. That was her plan, with very specific instructions from the get go.

She began writing letters by hand, almost as soon as she started researching ALS. She knew she would lose the ability to write and wanted so desperately for people to know what they meant to her. Never one to be without a plan, she wrote and shared her love of Jesus every day. She asked that each letter be placed in a basket alphabetically at the Celebration of Life Service.

She asked repeatedly if she had taken care of different tasks. She wrote hundreds of notes that became more difficult to read. She would nod if I had guessed correctly.

"Did I remember to mention I have clothes to donate to T.O.P.S?"

"Did we send a thank you note to Clara?"

"See if I wrote a letter to Ginger and Vern?"

"How is your blood sugar? You've got to take care of yourself. The boys need you."

It was always about everyone else. Not whether she was hurting or unable to breathe.

Every thought she shared was for others. She was so upset that she could not get up and serve others. She would write a note asking if I had offered visitors a Diet Coke. She liked for me to be there if someone was coming to visit because I could interpret her sign language or written notes more quickly than most people. One look with raised eyebrows, and I knew she needed her mouth wiped or her nails cleaned. She had always been the 'hostess with the moistest,' and now she could not make certain that people were at home in her home.

My husband, Chet would sit with her on Sunday mornings so Dad and I could go to church. That was the only time Dad would leave her side.

Mom would have a list for Chet. A list of things she wanted him to do. She would write me notes afterward saying what a blessing Chet was to our family. He has worked with the developmentally disabled for many years and would think of things the rest of us never considered. He set up a mirror when she could no longer turn her head, so that she could see people coming in through the back door. Chet created pen grips from foam that would make it easier for her to write. When she would get frustrated that no one understood what she wanted, she would finally say, "Get Chet, he'll know." I've never been so grateful to God for the amazing man that I married.

What do you want to be known for? Your love? Your generosity? Your talents? The lives you touched? The children you've left in the world? Making a difference?

She wanted her children, grandchildren and great-grandchildren to know and love the Lord Jesus Christ.

Her nephew, Gary Ashlock, read this prayer he wrote at her Celebration of Life Service:

Heavenly Father, Creator of the universe and everything within, we praise You. You are our rock, our hope, our salvation.

She was a wife, a mother, a grandmother, a sister, an aunt, a friend, a Christian.
She loved life and loved Jake, she loved her children; Dayna and Danice.

94

She loved her grandkids, she loved her sisters and brothers.

Gloria loved Jesus and the sacrifice He made for all of us. We praise His holy name.

We do not know why she had to leave us or why she had to suffer so long. We know

That You have called her to her heavenly home. We know that eternal life is only for

Those who do God's will. I know You are going to really enjoy Gloria. We are

Going to miss "Little Sister" so very much. We ask your Holy Spirit to comfort Jake and Dayna and Danice and all of her family and friends. We know Gloria doesn't hurt

Anymore and her eternal life has begun. Death to Christians is precious; Christians

Enter perfect peace at death. We do not know how long we will live; living in heaven is better than living on earth. Life comes from God and our lives should honor God.

Gloria honored God. God's love for us is beyond our understanding and we cannot be

Separated from Jesus' love. The Lord is my shepherd; I have everything I need. He leads

Me beside peaceful streams. He renews my strength. He guides me along right paths,

Bringing honor to his name.

Even when I walk through the dark valley of death, I will not be afraid for you are close beside me. Your rod and your staff protect and comfort me. You prepare a feast for me in the presence of my enemies. You welcome me as a guest, anointing my head with oil. My cup overflows with blessings. Surely your goodness and unfailing love will pursue me all the days of my life, and I will live in the house of the Lord forever. (Psalm 23)

In Christ holy name we pray. Amen

Let me paint you a picture of Gloria Clover: She wrote letters. Hundreds of letters. To friends, family, church members and loved ones. She shared her faith, her testimony and her love of the Lord. When she could no longer write because her hand "froze up" she would have Dad put splints on them, to try and keep her fingers from curling up. When the splints no longer worked, she would ask me to write for her.

We also used sign language, which we had both learned years before from a dear man, Gabriel Yankey, whom she adored.

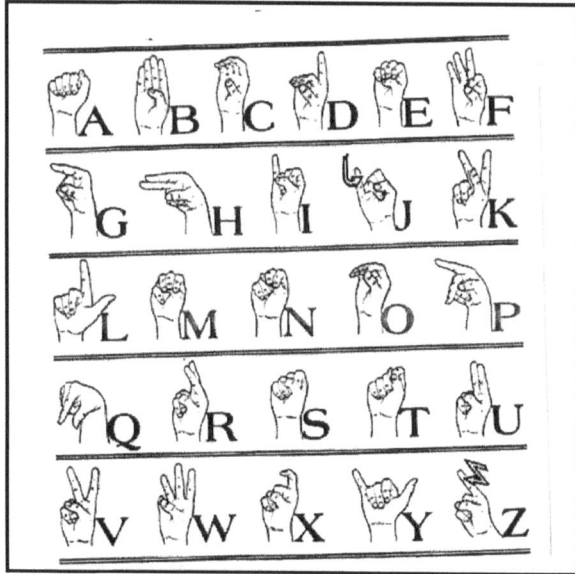

She believed that everyone should learn sign language. If you know the alphabet, you can at least spell something to anyone who is deaf. She had the cards printed up for people who came to visit, so they could understand what she would spell.

Before she was no longer able to sign, she also created a blinking system, similar to one she had seen on the internet. One blink for "yes" and two blinks for "no." Then there was the specific blinking system which we rehearsed in case that dreaded day came. Dividing the alphabet into thirds on a sheet of paper: A- J was one blink. K-R was 2 blinks and S-Z was 3 blinks. Once the row of thirds was selected the person holding the alphabet would go letter by letter to determine what she wanted to spell. It was a tiresome process but seemed like it might work.

She was very determined that I draw a paper doll so she could point to what hurt, when she could no longer write or sign. She could point or grab on to the place that hurt or needed adjusted.

Her feet would slide outward on her wheel chair, and the pressure would cause pain. Dad created and recreated all kinds of slings and pillows with elastic straps to hold her hand and keep it from falling. When her head would not stay up, and she could no longer control her neck muscles, we had a variety of pillows and splints and scarves. I never was a seamstress, my home economics teacher, Mrs. Bryant can attest to that, but when Mom wanted a long strip of foam to hold up her neck, I took some of her scarves and sewed them around the foam so the foam wouldn't scratch.

She started grinning when I brought in the first one. I asked her what was so funny, and she signed, "I didn't know you could sew!" Very aware of her appearance, she wanted the scarves to match her outfit. We had black ones that went with everything and a tiger stripe one on a copper background that matched her hair. (I have it in a Ziploc bag and it smells like my momma.)

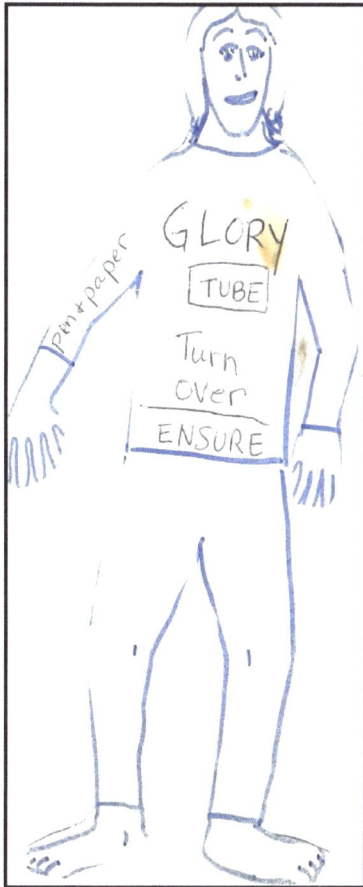

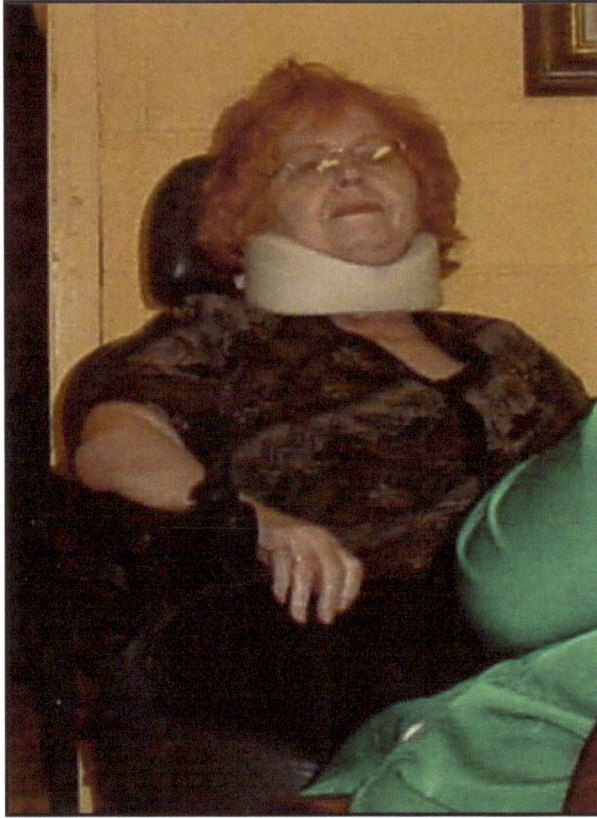

I saw on the Today Show, a woman with A.L.S. in her forties who had a neck brace that allowed air to still reach the skin around the neck. I searched for it on the computer and found it was called a cervical collar. I ordered one, and it arrived within the week and was a helpful alternative. Even it only helped for so long. Mom's body was disintegrating so fast that we could hardly keep up. As soon as we found something that worked, a new challenge presented itself. For example; once the neck braces made of a sponge-like foam started working, we had to watch very closely or her chin would sink down, covering her nose and mouth and preventing breathing. Dad created braces and brackets, lifts and slings, anything that would make her comfortable.

For a while she could eat her favorite thing, guacamole. Then she could only swallow a bite, then it would make her cough and gag and choke. Eventually a feeding tube was put in her stomach. Sometimes the liquid protein we gave her would come back up so quickly that we had to keep a towel on her chest. It was awful, seeing her struggle with everything from picking up a pen to signing I love you. The great-grandsons always ended each visit with a hug with Grammy and an "I love you" sign.

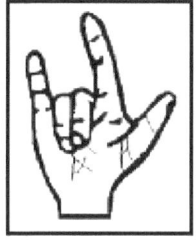

As my niece, Holly, picked up her boys from my house the other day, Gabriel said, "Wait, Nene." And showed me the "I love you" sign. I tried not to cry, because it reminded me of my momma. Now it's a symbol we always use with great love and affection.

The waves of sorrow come over me now like hurricane force winds leaving only devastation in their wake. I can't seem to get past the hurting. Hers or mine. She would ask me to scratch the nape of her neck or massage her shoulders or scratch her nose.

My mother, who taught children to read, who received her Doctor's degree in Theology, who organized banquets for the elderly, parties for children and concerts for everyone, could no longer reach up and wipe her nose or turn the page in a book. Her nieces and nephews got together and bought her a Kindle. A device from Amazon.com that allows you to download books and even reads them to you. She loved it. She would listen to positive books over and over.

A dear friend, Julie Kratt, came over every week to read to Mom. She was comforting and placed scriptures she had written out by hand, where Mom could see them. Julie had lost both her parents and has the wisdom and love for the Lord that shines out from her. She was a blessing to Mom and to our family. When you go through something like this together, there is a bond that lasts forever.

At Mom's Celebration of Life service, a dear friend and sister in Christ, Dianne Flickinger shared the following:

"Gloria challenged our group of ladies to go out and do random acts of kindness for others. Next thing I knew, I found two or three stick horses on my front porch for my three young children from someone who cared about others. My husband Mark found himself teaching Art Smart in several elementary schools and frequently visited Gloria's second grade classroom. The activity involved the use of crayons and Mark commented on how he always wanted a box of 64 crayons with a sharpener on the side when he was a child, but he never got it because it was too extravagant to have that many crayons. Later that same day, he found a box of 64 crayons with a sharpener on the side at the front door of our house. A lesson learned and a prize.

Jake and Gloria moved north of town to where they live now, and the church was invited to their place for food, fun, and fellowship. There was ping pong, air hockey, foosball, card tables, couches and a huge screen TV for all to enjoy! Many families from the church would come, and we spent time getting to know others from the church. Gloria always had a game with a lesson learned and prizes.

Then Gloria came up with the M.A.G.I.C. group - Most Active Group in Church for ages 50 and up. They would meet regularly, eat meals together, plan a Valentine's dinner for the church family, travel, and provide service projects for others. This group continues to make Christmas sacks for the children each year and an Easter activity involving eggs, candy and coins each spring. How often do you see the older and the younger getting to know one another at church? A lesson learned and prizes.

Our church supports Family Life Services in our community, and we have gone to clean their building and stuff envelopes on occasion, but now Gloria suggested that our Sunday School offering go to pay for sonograms to prevent pregnant women in our community from having an abortion. Our class has paid for at least seven sonograms to date. I made a point to bring more offering to Sunday School than I would have if Gloria had not given a direct purpose to our giving. When a church member had a financial need that we were aware of, the offering would go directly to them. Gloria taught us how to give. A lesson learned and a prize (only now I am beginning to realize that the prize is an internal reward in my heart).

God brought Jake and Gloria Clover to Bible Christian Church at a time when our church needed to experience and learn about hospitality. Gloria has been such a blessing to our church family. She always had a new idea of how to bring people together, show kindness, learn a lesson, and give a prize.

Gloria was elected to be President of our women's group for one year. We were just getting to know Gloria when she made us want to read the Bible and come each month for a meeting. She wanted us to read only one chapter each day for an entire month and then at the next meeting she would have a quiz. She typed out the entire chapter and left blanks for us to fill in the missing words. It was not easy if you did not read your chapter. Then we found out that there was a prize for the one who had the most correct answers. It was a new challenge that caused me to read more often throughout the week. A lesson learned and a prize.

It was time for a new Sunday School class in our new building called Faith Cafe. A sign made of colorful felt went up, coasters, index cards for prayer requests, a welcome sign, pencils, a Bible, Kleenex, and an offering container all went in the center of each table in the class so that everyone who came was thought of. Next thing you know, she had talked her daughter Danice into making a painting for the class. Breakfast snacks, coffee, and ice tea have been provided every Sunday since the beginning of this class and the class is still going on with Jake as our teacher. We have shed many a tear and have prayed for one another in this class. Most importantly, the very class that Jake and Gloria provided for others became a place of strength for them during this time of Gloria's illness. You see how God has used Gloria and her spiritual gifts to bring people together today, learn another lesson, and give more prizes (red-headed doll collection) even at her own funeral? God has used Gloria to teach our church family about bringing people together, showing kindness, learning a lesson, and giving a prize. She even told Danice to ask me to say a few words today, that in my sorrow and fear of crying, I may not have shared with you today." (used by permission.)

Why would the God of Heaven allow this to happen? I questioned my faith for the first time in my life. Cancer, diabetes and a heart attack, had not caused me to ask God why. But my mother's illness did. Those horrible letters "A. L. S." did.

That's not what she would want, but that's how it feels. Last night, my husband Chet said, "She would not want you spending one minute grieving over her, while she is rejoicing in Heaven with Jesus Christ and waiting for you to get there."

It's been one year since my mom went home to be with the Lord and everyday I feel the loss. Her letter to me said,

"...I just wanted you to have it in writing how much I love you and appreciate all your efforts to help me live, but it wasn't to be. I will live

forever though, and that's the only thing that is important. Don't waste time grieving about me.... Love you more than you'll ever know." Mom

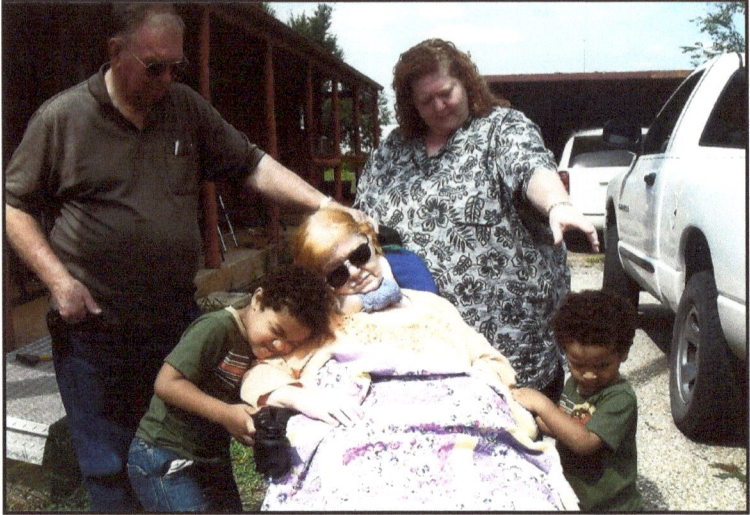

Left to right: Dad, Gabriel, Mom, Me, Noah.

I hesitated to include this photo. It's one of the last ones we have. You can see the pain in everyone's face except my mother's. She's ready to go home.

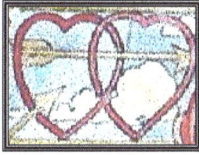

Chapter Fourteen: Her Hope

Mom is the most inspiring woman I've ever known. She was a life-long learner. Her faith continues to inspire people all over the world. When she went on to glory, November 9, 2009, she was ready to meet the Lord Jesus Christ. She wanted everyone else to be ready as well. We believe Jesus is the son of the Living God. We believe you need to be baptized for the remission of your sins. (Acts 2:38) We believe you need to walk the walk and talk the talk. It doesn't mean you are perfect, just forgiven.

In Mom's Checklist of Life, I found this paper folded in the back cover today.

LIFE PURPOSE STATEMENT OF

Gloria Ann (Hardy) Clover

WRITTEN _Dec. 15_ , 2006

1. **What will be the center of my life? (a question of worship)** _Serving Jesus as Lord and Savior._

2. **What will be the character of my life? (a question of discipleship)** _I hope people can see Jesus in my life._

3. **What will be the contribution of my life? (a question of service)** _I want to be an encourager through example of words and deeds._

4. **What will be the communication of my life? (a question of my mission to unbelievers)** _God is our creator and His son died for us and because of this great love and sacrifice by accepting Jesus as savior, and following we can have eternal life._

5. **What will be the community of my life? (a question of fellowship)** _I believe assembling and fellowship with like believers is very important and strengthens them and self._

EXAMPLES:

"My goal is Christlikeness; my family is the church; my ministry is _encouraging_; my mission is _to glorify the Lord_; my motive is the glory of God."
Or
"My life purpose is to worship Christ with my heart, serve him with my shape, fellowship with his family, grow like him in character, and fulfill his mission in the world so he receives glory."
Or
"My life purpose is to be a member of Christ's family, a model of his character, a minister of his grace, a messenger of his word, and a magnifier of his glory"
Or
"My life purpose is to love Christ, grow in Christ, share Christ, and serve Christ through his church, and to lead my family and others to do the same."
Or
"My life purpose is to make a great commitment to the Great Commandment and the Great Commission."

I want also want to encourage people to be baptized as it signifies the death, burial, and resurrection of Jesus whose sacrifices is our hope of eternal life

104

One of Mom's last requests was that Dad and I work on an ALS (Lou Gehrig's Disease) book for Christians. There just aren't any out there. Last Sunday morning, during church, God spoke to my heart. This may be the last chapter, or a start but since we're not sending out Christmas cards, I share this with you:

That day something changed. My mother, my model, my mentor went from this world to another place. I was there to see it. It was glorious for Gloria went on to glory. ALS had bound her feet, her legs, her arms and her head, but it could not bind her heart and soul. They were free to fly to Jesus. And how they flew! Without hesitation, without regret, she flew. As fast as angels can arrive by your side, she went to the streets of gold. One moment, one breath, and that veil was torn between the physical and the eternal. All her hope and dreams and prayers of relief arrived...completely healed and without pain, no longer sorrowful or strained. Christmas will be different this year, and we're all trying to adjust. For the one that made it special at our house is celebrating already in Heaven. She's enjoying the Savior's birth with the greatest gift ever: not a tree, or even a star, but the gift itself, Christ Jesus.

I think she would want everyone to know what she felt was her purpose here on earth. She fought the good fight, and finished the race.

As I think of her last day here on earth, a smile comes over my face. I remember a life well-lived, a faith fulfilled, a battle fought, and amazing satisfaction knowing

Gloria won.

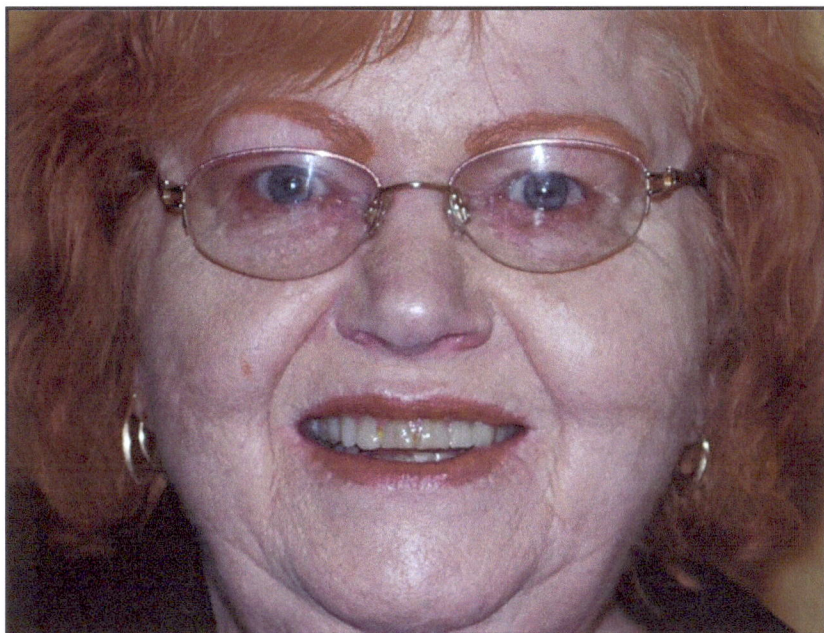

Bibliography

American Heart Organization (www.American heart.org) *Questions and Answers about Chelation Therapy.*

Amyotrophic lateral sclerosis fact sheet. National Institute of NeurologicalDisordersandStroke.http://www.nindsnih.gov/disorders/ amyotrophiclateralsclerosis/detail_amyotrophiclateralsclerosis.htm. Accessed Sept. 18, 2008.

Benefit Focus Media. http://www.icyou.com/topics/als-lou-gehrig-s-disease/what-amyotrophic-lateral-sclerosis-als+, (2010)

Edney, Eric, *Eric Is Winning: Beating a Terminal Illness with Nutrition, Avoiding Toxins and Common Sense.* (2004)

Flickinger, Dianne. *From Gloria Clover's Celebration of Life Service,* (Nov.2009)

Mayo Foundation for Medical Education and Research (MFMER). http://www.mayoclinic.com/health/amyotrophic-lateral-sclerosis/DS00359 (1998-2010).

McPhelimy, Lynn. *Checklist of Life*, p. 55, 67. (2007)

Mitsumoto, Hiroshi. *Amyotrophic Lateral Sclerosis: A Guide for Patients and Families.* (2009)

New International Version of the Holy Bible. Acts 2:38; Galatians 2:20; Luke 12:27; Mathew 6:27; Psalms 23, 89:4; Proverbs31.

Rouzier, Neal, http: Holisticonline.com/chelation/hol_chelation.htm (copyright1998-2007 ICBS) www.ericiswinning.com/about.html

Rylant, Cynthia and Stephen Gammell 1993. *The Relative Came.* Simon & Schuster Children's Publishing.

Stewart, Imogene. *The Glory Glow*. 2008. Shown courtesy of the author.

Newest ALS Research @www.physorg.com as of 9-13-10

Wikipedia. *Little House on the Prairie*. (en.wikipedia.org/wiki/Little House. 2010.

Pearson Publishing Company
Corpus Christi, Texas

For a complete list and description of our publications and to order books, please go to our website: www.PearsonPub.US

Saga of a Comanche Warrior
By Max Oliver
Book One: Little Boy $12.95
Book Two: No More $9.95
Book Three: Tomo Pui $9.95
Book Four: Red Nose $9.95
Book Five: Chief Red Nose $10.95

Slumbertime: A Parent's Guide for Children's Sleep and Sleep Problems $29.95
By Janet S. Gould
Catching the Dream: A Parent's Guide for Children's Dreams $26.95
By Janet S. Gould

Deal Me In $23.95
By Alyce Guynn with illustrations by Jesse Taylor

His Angels Are In Charge $24.95
By Frances Cotten Woodard

Floating Zoo and the Whale Motel $26.95
Written and illustrated by Danice Sweet
Consider It Joy $16.95
Written and illustrated by Danice Sweet
I Will Speak Your Name $16.95
Written and Illustrated by Danice Sweet
He Makes Me Laugh $21.95
Written and Illustrated by Danice Sweet

To mail in orders, send (1) a list of titles with number of copies of each title,
(2) check or money order for total retail price of all books,
plus (3) $5.00 shipping and handling for each book,
plus (4) your name and mailing address printed clearly, to:

Pearson Publishing Company
555 S. Shoreline Blvd., Suite 104
Corpus Christi, Texas 78401

www.ingramcontent.com/pod-product-compliance
Lightning Source LLC
Chambersburg PA
CBHW040130270326
41928CB00001B/13